AF443423

RECENT ADVANCES IN THE EPIDEMIOLOGY AND PREVENTION OF GALLSTONE DISEASE

Developments in Gastroenterology

VOLUME 12

RECENT ADVANCES IN THE EPIDEMIOLOGY AND PREVENTION OF GALLSTONE DISEASE

Proceedings of the Second International Workshop on Epidemiology and Prevention of Gallstone Disease, held in Rome, December 4—5, 1989

edited by

L. Capocaccia, G. Ricci, F. Angelico, M. Angelico, A. F. Attili and L. Lalloni

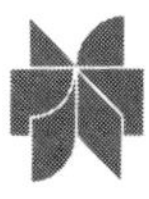

KLUWER ACADEMIC PUBLISHERS
DORDRECHT / BOSTON / LONDON

Library of Congress Cataloging-in-Publication Data

```
International Workshop on the Epidemiology and Prevention of Gallstone
   Disease (2nd : 1989 : Rome Italy)
   Recent advances in the epidemiology and prevention of gallston
 disease : proceedings of the second International Workshop on
 Epidemiology and Prevention of Gallstone Disease / edited by L.
 Capocaccia ... [et. al.].
       p.   cm. -- (Development in gastroenterology ; 12)
   Includes index.
   ISBN 0-7923-0994-4 (alk. paper)
   1. Gallstones--Epidemiology--Congresses.  2. Gallstones-
 -Prevention--Congresses.   I. Cappocaccia, Livio.  II. Title.
 III. Series.
   [DNLM: 1. Cholelithiasis--epidemiology--congresses.
 2. Cholelithiasis--prevention & control--congresses.  3. Risk
 Factors--congresses.   W1 DE997VYB v. 12 / WI 755 I593r 1989]
 RA645.G34I58  1989
 614.5'9365--dc20
 DNLM/DLC
 for Library of Congress                                 90-5388
```

ISBN 0-7923-0994-4

Published in the United Kingdom by Kluwer Academic Publishers,
P.O. Box 55, Lancaster, United Kingdom

Kluwer Academic Publishers incorporates
the publishing programmes of
D. Reidel, Martinus Nijhoff, Dr W. Junk and MTP Press.

Sold and distributed in the U.S.A. and Canada
by Kluwer Academic Publishers,
101 Philip Drive, Norwell, MA 02061, U.S.A.

In all other countries, sold and distributed
by Kluwer Academic Publishers Group,
P.O. Box 322, 3300 AH Dordrecht, The Netherlands.

Printed on acid-free paper

Printed in The Netherlands

Table of contents

List of contributors

M. ACALOVSCHI, IIIrd Medical Clinic, Department of Gastroenterology, Cluj-Napoca, Romania.

G. AGNELLO, Department of Gynaecology, V. Cervello Hospital, Palermo, Italy.

V. ALVISI, Institute of Clinical Medicine, University of Ferrara, Ferrara, Italy.

F. ANGELICO, Institute of Systematical Medical Therapy, University of Rome 'La Sapienza', Rome, Italy.

M. ANGELICO, 2nd Department of Gastroenterology, University of Rome 'La Sapienza', Rome, Italy.

A.F. ATTILI, Gastroenterology Unit, Department of Internal Medicine, University of L'Aquila, L'Aquila, Italy.

P. BACCELLIERE, Medical Clinic 'R', V. Cervello Hospital, Palermo, Italy.

R. BADEA, IIIrd Medical Clinic, Department of Gastroenterology, Cluj-Napoca, Romania.

C. BANTERLE, Department of General Medicine, Ospedale di Desenzano, Desenzano, Italy.

L. BARBARA, Institute of Clinical Medicine and Gastroenterology, University of Bologna, Bologna, Italy.

L. BARRESI, Medical Clinic 'R', V. Cervello Hospital, Palermo, Italy.

M.C. BATESON, Department of Gastroenterology, General Hospital, Bishop Auckland, County Durham, DL14 6AP, United Kingdom.

D. BLENDEA, IIIrd Medical Clinic, Department of Gastroenterology, Cluj-Napoca, Romania.

G.G. BONORRIS, Division of Gastroenterology, Cedars-Sinai Medical Center and UCLA, Los Angeles, CA, U.S.A.

P.H. BROOMFIELD, Division of Gastroenterology, Cedars-Sinai Medical Center and UCLA, Los Angeles, CA, U.S.A.

L. CAPOCACCIA, 2nd Department of Gastroenterology, University of Rome 'La Sapienza', Rome, Italy.

R. CAPRI, Gastroenterology Unit, Department of Internal Medicine, University of L'Aquila, L'Aquila, Italy.

M. CIAMBRA, Medical Clinic 'R', V. Cervello Hospital, Palermo, Italy.

S. COLASANTI, Institute of Clinical Medicine and Gastroenterology, Department of General Medicine, Ospedale di Desenzano, University of Bologna, Bologna, Italy.

G.L. CORNIA, Institute of Clinical Medicine and Gastroenterology, University of Bologna, Bologna, Italy.

A. DE SANTIS, 2nd Department of Gastroenterology, University of Rome 'La Sapienza', Rome, Italy.

A.K. DIEHL, Division of General Medicine, Department of Medicine, University of Texas Health Science Center, San Antonio, TX 78284-7879, U.S.A.

D. FESTI, Institute of Clinical Medicine and Gastroenterology, University of Bologna, Bologna, Italy.

G. FORMENTINI, Institute of Clinical Medicine and Gastroenterology, Department of General Medicine, Ospedale di Desenzano, University of Bologna, Bologna, Italy.

R. FRABBONI, Institute of Clinical Medicine and Gastroenterology, Department of General Medicine, Ospedale di Desenzano, University of Bologna, Bologna, Italy.

G.D. FRIEDMAN, Division of Research, Kaiser Permanente Medical Care Program, Northern California Region, Oakland, CA 94611, U.S.A.

A. GEORECEANU, IIIrd Medical Clinic, Department of Gastroenterology, Cluj-Napoca, Romania.

T. GILAT, Department of Gastroenterology, Ichilov Hospital, Tel Aviv, Israel.

S. GINNANI CORRADINI, 2nd Department of Gastroenterology, University of Rome 'La Sapienza', Rome, Italy.

E.P. GIULIANI, 2nd Department of Gastroenterology, University of Rome 'La Sapienza', Rome, Italy.

R. GRASSO, Medical Clinic 'R', V. Cervello Hospital, Palermo, Italy.

D. GULLO, Department of Gynaecology, V. Cervello Hospital, Palermo, Italy.

Z. HALPERN, Department of Gastroenterology, Ichilov Hospital, Tel Aviv, Israel.

R.M. IEMMOLO, Institute of Internal Medicine, University Clinic, Padova, Italy.

N. IKEDA, Self-Defence Forces Fukuoka Hospital, Fukuoka, Japan.

K. IMANISHI, Self-Defence Forces Fukuoka Hospital, Fukuoka, Japan.

S. KONO, Department of Public Health, Fukuoka University School of Medicine Nanakuma, Fukuoka, Japan.

L. LALLONI, Institute of Systematical Medical Therapy, University of Rome 'La Sapienza', Rome, Italy.

F. LIRUSSI, Institute of Internal Medicine, University Clinic, Padova, Italy.

A. MARINGHINI, Medical Clinic 'R', V. Cervello Hospital, Palermo, Italy.

J.W. MARKS, Division of Gastroenterology, Cedars-Sinai Medical Center and UCLA, Los Angeles, CA, U.S.A.

S. MASELLI, Gastroenterology Unit, Department of Internal Medicine, University of L'Aquila, L'Aquila, Italy.

C.K. McSHERRY, Department of Surgery, Beth Israel Medical Center, New York, NY 10003, U.S.A.

A. MENOTTI, Istituto Superiore di Sanità, Laboratory of Epidemiology and Biostatistics, Rome, Italy.

O. MORENI, Institute of Clinical Medicine and Gastroenterology, Department of General Medicine, Ospedale di Desenzano, University of Bologna, Bologna, Italy.

A.M. MORSELLI LABATE, Institute of Clinical Medicine and Gastroenterology, University of Bologna, Bologna, Italy.

M.C. NACCHIERO, Institute of Clinical Medicine and Gastroenterology, University of Bologna, Bologna, Italy.

F. NARDIN, Institute of Clinical Medicine and Gastroenterology, University of Bologna, Bologna, Italy.

G. NASSUATO, Institute of Internal Medicine, University Clinic, Padova, Italy.

L. OKOLICSANYI, Institute of Internal Medicine, University Clinic, Padova, Italy.

A. ORLANDO, Medical Clinic 'R', V. Cervello Hospital, Palermo, Italy.

L. PAGLIARO, Medical Clinic 'R', V. Cervello Hospital, Palermo, Italy.

S. PARRO, Institute of Clinical Medicine and Gastroenterology, University of Bologna, Bologna, Italy.

D. PASSERA, Institute of Internal Medicine, University Clinic, Padova, Italy.

P. PAZZI, 1st Medical Division, Arcispedale S. Anna, Ferrara, Italy.

M.C. PILIA, Institute of Clinical Medicine and Gastroenterology, University of Bologna, Bologna, Italy.

G. POLLINI, Institute of Clinical Medicine and Gastroenterology, University of Bologna, Bologna, Italy.

A. PUCI, Institute of Clinical Medicine and Gastroenterology, University of Bologna, Bologna, Italy.

M. RAIMONDO, Medical Clinic 'R', V. Cervello Hospital, Palermo, Italy.

M. RANDAZZO, Medical Clinic 'R', V. Cervello Hospital, Palermo, Italy.

A.M. REPICE, Gastroenterology Unit, Department of Internal Medicine, University of L'Aquila, L'Aquila, Italy.

G. RICCI, Institute of Systematical Medical Therapy, University of Rome 'La Sapienza', Rome, Italy.

E. RODA, Institute of Clinical Medicine and Gastroenterology, University of Bologna, Bologna, Italy.

M. ROSSI, Institute of Clinical Medicine and Gastroenterology, University of Bologna, Bologna, Italy.

A.G. RUSTICALI, Institute of Clinical Medicine and Gastroenterology, University of Bologna, Bologna, Italy.

C. SAMA, Institute of Clinical Medicine and Gastroenterology, University of Bologna, Bologna, Italy.

S. SAMMARCO, Medical Clinic 'R', V. Cervello Hospital, Palermo, Italy.

L.J. SCHOENFIELD, Division of Gastroenterology, Cedars-Sinai Medical Center and UCLA, Los Angeles, CA, U.S.A.

D. SIGHINOLFI, Institute of Clinical Medicine, University of Ferrara, Ferrara, Italy.

K. SHINCHI, Self-Defence Forces Fukuoka Hospital, Fukuoka, Japan.

J. STAMLER, Department of Community Health and Preventive Medicine, Northwestern University Medical School, Chicago, IL, U.S.A.

F. TARONI, Istituto Superiore di Sanità, Laboratory of Epidemiology and Biostatistics, Rome, Italy.

G. TASSINARI, Institute of Clinical Medicine and Gastroenterology, University of Bologna, Bologna, Italy.

F. TINÈ, Medical Clinic 'R', V. Cervello Hospital, Palermo, Italy.

S. TOSO, Institute of Internal Medicine, University Clinic, Padova, Italy.

M. YAMAMOTO, Self-Defence Forces Fukuoka Hospital, Fukuoka, Japan.

F. YANAI, Self-Defence Forces Fukuoka Hospital, Fukuoka, Japan.

Composition of the Rome group of 'Epidemiology and Prevention of Cholelithiasis' (GREPCO)

Chairman: L. Capocaccia (1979—90), Ricci (1979—90).

Steering Committee: F. Angelico (1979—90), M. Angelico (1979—90), A.F. Attili (1979—90).

Coordination: A. Calvieri (1979—84), P. Clemente (1979—83), A. De Santis (1979—90), L. Lalloni (1979—90), G. Morisi (1979—90), G.C. Urbinati (1982—84).

Clinical Staff: D. Alvaro (1979—84), L. Antonaci (1983—84), A. Cantagalli (1987—88), R. Capri (1985—89), S. Cocca (1981—84), M. Colzi (1980—84), M. Del Ben (1984—88), F. Gianbenedetti (1987—88), S. Ginanni Corradini (1987—88), S. Gualandi (1987—88), P. Guccione (1979—81), M. Marin (1982—84), S. Maselli (1989—90), P. Monini (1979—82), L. Massa (1983—84), P. Pallotto (1987—88), A.M. Repice (1989—90), G. Rimenti (1987—88), C. Stefanutti (1982—88), E. Scafato (1980—90), A. Scarno (1987—88).

Echographic and Radiologic Staff: L. Azzarri (1987—88), R. Conti (1982—88), L. Lalloni (1979—90), F. Mariucci (1980—81), D. Minasi (1984), P. Ricci (1984—88), M. Valeo (1987—88).

Biochemical Staff: M. Arca (1980—87), A. Buongiorno (1980—85), S. Ciocca (1981—84), S. Fazio (1983—85), A. Montali (1980—87), G. Morisi (1979—90), U. Pieche (1979—82), A. Zucca (1981—82).

Biostatistical Staff: Fa. Angelico (1979—82), A. Calvieri (1979—83), R. Capocaccia (1979—90), A. Menotti (1979—90), R. Scipione (1983—84).

Editorial Board: F. Angelico (1979—90), M. Angelico (1979—90), M. Arca (1983—90), A.F. Attili (1979—90), L. Capocaccia (1979—90), G. Ricci (1979—90).

Acknowledgement

We would like to thank Joan Crowley, B.A., for revising the English text.

Composition of research group: Italian multicentre study on epidemiology and prevention of cholelithiasis (MICOL)

Centre of Bari
   III Clinica Medica, Università di Bari
   Directors: O. Albano, G. Palasciano
   Principal Investigators: G. Calò Gabrieli, P. Portincasa, S. Tardi
   Biochemical Staff: G. Vendemiale, A. Velardi
   Field Staff: V. Vinciguerra, G. Baldassarre, C. Origlia, V. Palmieri, N. Morelli, A. Belfiore

Centre of Bologna I
   Clinica Medica III, Policlinico S. Orsola, Universita' di Bologna
   Director: L. Barbara
   Principal investigator: E. Roda
   Biochemical staff: M.S. Benassi, M. Forni
   Field staff: D. Festi, R. Frabboni, A.M. Morselli-Labate, M.C. Nacchiero, S. Parro, G. Pollini, M. Rossi, A.G. Rusticali, C. Sama, G. Tassinari, G. Cane', B. Crino', O. Masiello, D. Panuccio, A. Romani, R. Romanelli

Centre of Bologna II
   Cattedra di Gerontologia, Universita' di Bologna
   Director: Prof. G.C. Descovich
   Principal investigators: A. Dormi, G.L. Magri
   Biochemical staff: Z. Sangiorgi, G. Copparoni, C. La Regina, C. Meotti
   Field staff: B. Benassi, M.L. Borlotti, A. Cavina, M. Ceccardi, C. Ceredi, S. D'Addato, B. Descovich, C. Descovich, G. De Simone, E. Faggioli, A. Gaddi, A. Minardi, A. Matteucci, G. Negro, S. Rimondi, G.B. Sisca, D. Vici, M. Vigna

Centre of Bolzano
   Divisione di Gastroenterologia, Ospedale Generale Regionale, Bolzano
   Director: G. Dobrilla
   Principal investigators; M. Valentini, G. De Pretis
   Biochemical staff: U. Gaspa
   Field staff: S. Amplatz, S. Benvenuti, I. Bresolin

Centre of Cagliari
   Divisione di Medicina Interna, Centro per la lotta contro l'Arterio sclerosi, Ospedale Brotzu, Cagliari

Director: S. Muntoni
Principal investigator: F. Pintus
Biochemical staff: F. Pintus
Field staff: P. Pintus, P. Mascia, E. Ganga, R. Ganga, P. Tronci, G. Cabiddu

Centre of Castellana Grotte
Ospedale Spec. in Gastroenterologia, IRCCS, Castellana Grotte
Director: I. Giorgio
Principal investigator: G. Misciagna
Biochemical staff: C. Messa, V. Mangini
Field staff: G. Angelelli, S. Elba, A. Mossa, M. Noviello, J. Petruzzi

Centre of Como
Divisione di Medicina Interna, Ospedale di Niguarda, Milano
Director: G. Ideo
Principal investigators: G. Ideo, B. Caspani
Biochemical staff: M. Cavalleri
Field staff: B. Caspani, A. Molteni, A. Stefini, G.B. Molteni, D. Albonico, G. Alfieri, D. Gola, M. Guanziroli, G. Carrara, L. Snider, G. Restelli

Centre of Ferrara
Istituto di Clinica Medica, Università di Ferrara e I° Divisione Medicina Arcispedale S. Anna, Ferrara
Director: V. Alvisi
Principal investigator: P. Pazzi
Biochemical staff: G. Guerra, D. Franzè
Field staff: F. Pavani, M. Massari, S. Putinati, M. Vincenzi, A. Laterza, D. Ferraresi, I. Caberletti, C. Andreati, L. Trevisani, G. Bozzolani, A. Zangirolami, D. Sighinolfi, G. Stabellini, A. D'Ambrosi.

Centre of Firenze
Istituto Clinica Medica IV, Universita' di Firenze
Director: P. Gentilini
Principal investigators: G. Buzzelli, F. Curradi
Biochemical staff: C. Ignesti
Field staff: P. Bandini, L. La Villa, U. Arena, C. Smorlesi, C. Bonechi, D. Coletta, D. Mondanelli, G. Parronchi, L. Mondelli, E. Calabrese

Centre of Milano
Clinica Medica III, Universita' di Milano
Director: M. Podda
Principal investigator: M. Zuin
Biochemical staff: U. Alieri

Field staff: P.M. Battezzati, E. Bertolini, A. Crosignani, C. De Fazio, G. Grandinetti, A. Camisasca, C. Caserta, M.L. Petroni, P. Roccucci

Centre of Modena I
  Istituto Clinica Medica I, Universita' di Modena
  Director: N. Carulli
  Principal investigators: P. Loria, D. Menozzi
  Biochemical staff: G. Grossi
  Field staff: G. Medici, A. Tripodi, L. Roncucci, M. Montanari, P. Di Donato, M. Iori, A. Digrisolo, R. Iori, V. Boraldi, D. Gollini, C. Sacche

Centre of Modena II
  Istituto Clinica Medica, Universita' di Modena
  Director: G. Salvioli
  Principal investigator: R. Lugli
  Biochemial staff: A. Carbonieri, E. Gaetti
  Field staff: G. Nasi, E. Tondelli, V. Boccaletti, A. Frignani, J. Pradelli

Centre of Napoli
  Istituto Medicina Interna e Malattie Metaboliche, II Facolta', Universita' di Napoli
  Director: M. Mancini
  Principal investigators: E. Farinaro, F. Contaldo
  Biochemical staff: G. De Biase.
  Field staff: N. Maturo, A. Cecere, G. Fusco, G. Di Biase

Centre of Padova
  Istituto Medicina Interna, Universita' di Padova
  Directors: L. Okolicsanyi, G. Crepaldi
  Principal investigators: A. Burlina, C. Zacchi, G. Rampazzo
  Biochemical staff: G. De Franchis, N. Di Vitofrancesco
  Field staff: G. Nassuato, F. Angelini, A. Fragasso, R.M. Iemmolo, M. Muraca, R. Orlando, D. Passera, M. Strazzabosco

Centre of Pietra Ligure
  Ospedale S. Corona, Divisione di Medicina Generale, Pietra Ligure
  Director: G. Marenco
  Principal investigator: G. Marenco
  Biochemical staff: L. Santorirella
  Field staff: P. Colombo, A. Artom, A. Giudici Cipriani, U. Folco

Centre of Roma I
  II Cattedra di Gastroenterologia, Clinica Medica III, Universita' di Roma 'La Sapienza'

    Director: L. Capocaccia
    Principal investigator: A.F. Attili
    Biochemical staff: G. Pinto
    Field staff: A. De Santis, S. Ginanni Corradini, C. De Luca, A. Romiti, E. Scafato, D. Porto, R. Capri, A. Cantagalli, E. Giuliani, F. Giambenedetti, A. Rosati, S. Gualandi, P. Pallotto

Centre of Roma II
    Istituto di Terapia Medica Sistematica, Universita' di Roma 'La Sapienza'
    Director: G. Ricci
    Principal investigator: L. Lalloni
    Biochemical staff: R. Antonini, R. Cantini, S. Ciocca, B. Mazzarella, F. Pacioni, A. Zucca
    Field staff: G. Argento, A. Azzarri, L. Azzarri, L. Bava, A. Bucci, R. Conti, I. De Felici, D. Degano, G. Graziani, L. Martini, A. Montali, P. Palombo, F. Pelliccia, G. Prosperi, B. Quattrini, P. Ricci, F. Ricciardi, G. Santoboni, A. Scarno, M. Valeo

Centre of Roma III
    Laboratorio di Epidemiologia e Biostatistica, Istituto Superiore di Sanita', Roma
    Director: A. Menotti
    Principal investigators: R. Capocaccia, S. Mariotti, F. Taroni, F. Valente

Centre of Roma IV
    Laboratorio di Biochimica Clinica, Istituto Superiore di Sanita', Roma
    Director: G. Morisi
    Principal investigator: G. Morisi
    Biochemical staff: A.M. Buongiorno

Centre of Verona
    Istituto Clinica Medica, Universita' di Verona
    Directors: L.A. Scuro, G. Angelini
    Principal investigator: G. Angelini
    Biochemical staff: M. Zatti
    Field staff: G. Antolini, A. Bonioli, E. Bottona, A. Castagnini, G. Degani, G. Di Stefano, A. Fratta Pasini, E. Lavarini, G. Montagnoli, S. Perbellini, G. Pisani, L. Rigo, P. Rizzini, T. Sandrini, M. Sciortino, N. Tallon, D. Zordan

PART ONE

Methodology, prevalence and incidence of gallstone disease

1. The GREPCO studies: methodology, prevalence and incidence data

F. ANGELICO and THE ROME GROUP FOR EPIDEMIOLOGY
AND PREVENTION OF CHOLELITHIASIS (GREPCO)*

Ten years have elapsed since the Rome group for the Epidemiology and Prevention of Cholelithiasis (GREPCO) started its research activities on the study of the epidemiology of gallstone disease. At that time most of the available information was derived from autopsy and clinical series. The few epidemiological studies performed by oral cholecystectomy in representative samples of free-living subjects had been carried out in populations known to be at high risk for developing gallstones on account of possible genetic factors and no studies on the prevalence of silent gallstones had been performed. In addition, the causal role of possible risk factors had been evaluated in only a few prospective studies, which were not primarily devoted to the study of gallstones and where cases were mostly subjects already cholecystectomized.

The introduction, in the late 70s, of ultrasonography for the detection of gallstones markedly changed the approach to the study of the epidemiology of gallstones. In fact, it was now possible to perform risk-free epidemiological surveys on samples of the general population and also obtain information on the prevalence and occurrence of silent stones [1]. On the basis of these developments, the GREPCO research group was founded in 1980 with the following aims [2]:
— to detect the prevalence of symptomatic and silent gallstones in different free-living communities
— to identify factors associated with the disease
— to study the incidence of gallstone disease in gallstone-free population samples.
— to identify risk factors
— to carry out preventive programmes
— to organize meetings

Since that date, four different population samples have been studied, for a total of 1964 males and 1480 females. They include 1244 male and 1081 female civil servants in Rome [3—7], 399 women from the rural community

* For the composition of the GREPCO group see p. x (list of contributors).

L. Capocaccia et al. (eds), Recent advances in the epidemiology and prevention of gallstone disease, 3—6.
© 1991 *Kluwer Academic Publishers. Printed in the Netherlands.*

Table 1. The GREPCO studies.

1081 Female civil servants, Rome
baseline survey February 1981—April 1982
1st rescreening November 1987—April 1988

1239 Male civil servants, Rome
baseline survey December 1982—July 1984

399 Rural women, Sezze
baseline survey January 1985—June 1985
within the DISCO Community Control Project of
Chronic Diseases of the National Research Council

367 Men belonging to a preventive treatment group
358 Men belonging to a control group
baseline survey November 1983—April 1984
within the Rome Project of Coronary Heart Disease
Prevention — WHO Multifactor Preventive Trial of CHD

---

of Sezze, 100 km south of Rome [8], and two samples of 367 and 358 men enrolled as treatment and control groups in a multifactor preventive trial of ischemic heart disease [9] (Table 1).

In all the above studies screening operations included an ultrasound examination of the gallbladder, a questionnaire on history and clinical symptoms, a collection of blood samples and a physical examination. Greater detail on the echographic criteria for the assessment of gallbladder status, laboratory methods and other screening procedures have been given elsewhere [1, 3, 4].

In all studies the prevalence of gallstone disease increased with age (Table 2). Among civil servants, the prevalence of gallstone disease was higher in women, the male to female ratio being 1:2.9, 1:1.6 and 1:1.2 in subjects aged 30—39, 40—49 and 50—59 yr respectively, indicating that gallstone formation occurs at a younger age in women than in men. The very high prevalence of gallstone disease in men over 50 was indeed unexpected. The prevalence of gallstone disease was higher in rural women than that observed in the female civil servants, suggesting that differences in genetic, environmental and lifestyle characteristics have a role to play, as well as risk factor levels, in gallstone formation. The proportion of subjects who had had a cholecystectomy in the past was 36.2, 35.2 and 41.1% for male and female civil servants and rural women respectively. Subjects with symptomatic gallstones were defined as those non cholecystectomized, who during the last five years had suffered from an abdominal pain in the right epicondrium or epigastrium lasting more than half an hour. Men with gallstones were less frequently symptomatic than female civil servants and rural women (Table 3). Symptomatology was rather similar among female civil servants and rural

Table 2. Age-specific prevalence of gallstone disease (gallstones plus cholecystectomy in civil servants, Rome and in rural women, Sezze.

| Age groups | Civil servants, Rome | | Rural women, Sezze |
	males (n = 1244)	females (n = 1081)	(n = 399)
20—29	2.3	2.5	2.2
30—39	2.2	5.9	6.5
40—49	6.7	10.9	14.0
50—59	14.7	17.8	25.9
60—69	14.4	25.0	27.5

Table 3. Prevalence of biliary pain during the previous five years.

| Symptomatology | Civil servants, Rome | | Rural women, Sezze |
	males (n = 102)	females (n = 102)	(n = 68)
Biliary pain and cholecystectomy	36.3	36.4	41.2
Biliary pain and no cholecystectomy	4.9	23.2	10.3
No abdominal pain	58.8	40.4	48.5

women, suggesting a similar natural history of the disease in different communities.

The prevalence of the so-called 'minor' or dyspeptic symptoms did not appear to be correlated, either in males or in females, with the presence of gallstones.

The proportion of gallstone subjects unaware of their condition was highest among male civil servants (87.6%) as compared to female civil servants (66.7%) and rural women (72.5%).

Presence of biliary symptoms in the five years prior to the studies and awareness of having gallstones were not related to any radiologic feature in 82 of the gallstone subjects who underwent oral cholecystography [7].

The role of the substitution of saturated for unsaturated fat and the use of hypolipidaemic drugs was investigated in men, who participated as treatment or control groups in the Rome Project of Coronary Heart Disease Prevention, a six-year multifactor preventive trial of ischemic heart disease [9]. Three years after the end of the trial, the prevalence of subjects with gallstones was not significantly different between men belonging to treatment (7.3%) and control (9.6%) groups, although a higher proportion of men had undergone cholecystectomy in the group submitted to preventive treatment (8.3% versus 4.3%). However, a higher prevalence of gallstone disease was observed among 40 men, who received lipid lowering drugs (almost entirely represented by clofibrate) for at least six months (22.5% versus 14.2% in the remaining subjects).

Preliminary data on the incidence of gallstone disease were obtained in 720 gallstone-free female civil servants, who underwent a second ultrasound examination of the gallbladder six years after the baseline screening. In this sample, the incidence of gallstone disease was 3.5/1000/yr. Among new cases, 18.7% had received cholecystectomy, 31.3% had developed biliary pain, 6.2% had suffered from non-specific abdominal pain and 43.8% did not develop any symptomatology. In agreement with the above findings, only 31.3% of women were aware of having developed gallstone disease.

References

1. Lalloni L and the GREPCO Group (1984): Gallbladder ultrasonography as a diagnostic tool in epidemiological screenings, pp. 111—115 in Capocaccia L, Ricci G, Angelico F, Angelico M, Attili AF (eds), *Epidemiology and Prevention of Gallstone Disease* Lancaster: MTP Press Limited.
2. Ricci G and the GREPCO Group (1984): The GREPCO research programmes: aims and prevalence data, pp. 9—14 in Capocaccia L, Ricci G, Angelico F, Angelico M, Attili AF (eds), *Epidemiology and Prevention of Gallstone Disease* Lancaster: MTP Press Limited.
3. Rome Group for Epidemiology and Prevention of Cholelithiasis (GREPCO) (1982): Prevalenza della colelitiasi: osservazioni preliminari su un campione di popolazione lavorativa femminile. *Epatologia* 28: 79—88.
4. Rome Group for Epidemiology and Prevention of Cholelithiasis (GREPCO) (1984): Prevalence of gallstone disease in an Italian adult female population *Am J Epidemiol* 119: 796—805.
5. Rome Group for Epidemiology and Prevention of Cholelithiasis (GREPCO) (1988): The epidemiology of gallstone disease in Rome, Italy. Part 1. Prevalence data in men. *Hepatology* 8: 904—906.
6. Rome Group for Epidemiology and Prevention of Cholelithiasis (GREPCO) (1988): The epidemiology of gallstone disease in Rome, Italy. Part 2. Factors associated with the disease. *Hepatology* 8: 907—913.
7. Rome Group for Epidemiology and Prevention of Cholelithiasis (GREPCO) (1987): Radiologic appearance of gallstones and its relationship with biliary symptoms and awareness of having gallstones: observations during epidemiological studies. *Dig Dis Sci* 32: 349—353.
8. Rome Group for Epidemiology and Prevention of Cholelithiasis (GREPCO) (1987): Epidemiology of gallstone disease in Italy: comparison between a rural and urban female population. *It J Gastroenterol* 18: 129—133.
9. Urbinati GC and the GREPCO Group (1984): Prevention of coronary heart disease and risk of cholelithiasis, pp. 193—198 in Capocaccia L, Ricci G, Angelico F, Angelico M, Attili AF (eds), *Epidemiology and Prevention of Gallstone Disease* Lancaster: MTP Press Limited.

2. Prevalence and incidence of gallstone disease: the Sirmione study

D. FESTI, L. BARBARA, R. FRABBONI, A. M. MORSELLI LABATE,
M. C. NACCHIERO, S. PARRO, G. POLLINI, E. RODA, M. ROSSI,
A. G. RUSTICALI, C. SAMA, F. TARONI, G. TASSINARI,
C. FORMENTINI, O. MORENI, F. NARDIN,
M. C. PILIA, and A. PUCI

Introduction

Cholelithiasis is a very common, world-wide disease; however estimates of its frequency have been made for many years, in autopsy studies and in studies on clinically diagnosed gallstone cases [1—3]. These studies cannot give a real insight into the problem, because a large proportion of gallstones remains asymptomatic and therefore ignored for many years or even forever [4, 5].

Only prospective studies actively investigating on large population samples can therefore give a real estimate of the prevalence of gallstone disease. These studies, however, necessitate of a simple and non invasive technique for detecting gallstones; ultrasonography, beside having a high sensitivity and specificity compared with the traditional X-ray procedures, is simple, safe and non-invasive and, therefore, represents the ideal tool for these studies [6, 7].

Methods

In 1982 we decided to initiate a cohort study with the purpose of ascertain the incidence and risk factors of gallstone disease in a general population and we choose the town of Sirmione which is located on lake Garda in the North of Italy.

From the Municipal Census of Sirmione, all subjects aged 18 to 65 years were selected for the study.

The screening protocol included a questionnaire, an ultrasonographic examination of the upper abdomen, a physical examination and a blood sample taken in the fasting condition. The precoded questionnaire included social and demographic data, medical and family history, and dietary habit. Part of the questionnaire inquired as to the presence of both specific and non specific biliary symptoms. More details on the study have been published elsewhere [8].

L. Capocaccia et al. (eds), Recent advances in the epidemiology and prevention of gallstone disease, 7—11.
© 1991 *Kluwer Academic Publishers. Printed in the Netherlands.*

Ultrasonography was performed using a real time machine (Aloka SSD-202) with a 3.5 MHz linear transducer. Overnight fasting subjects were studied in supine, left lateral and standing positions consecutively, and, in order to define cases of cholelithiasis, the following ultrasonographic pictures were selected [9]:

1. one or more echogenic, possible movable, distally shadowing structures within the gallbladder;
2. one or more echogenic, possible movable, nonshadowing structures within the gallbladder;
3. high-density echoes and constant shadowing in the region of the gallbladder fossa, with poor or no visualization of the gallbladder itself; and
4. one or more echogenic structures, with or without acoustic shadowing, within the biliary tree.

Results

Of the total population asked to participate (2732 persons), 1930 (70.6%) entered the study. Acceptance rates were slightly higher in women ($P < 0.01$) and increased steadily with age ($P < 0.001$) (Fig. 1).

The first cross sectional study was completed at the end of 1982.

The overall prevalence of gallstone disease was 11% (Table 1); 132 subjects had gallstones in their gallbladder at the time of the study (6.9%)

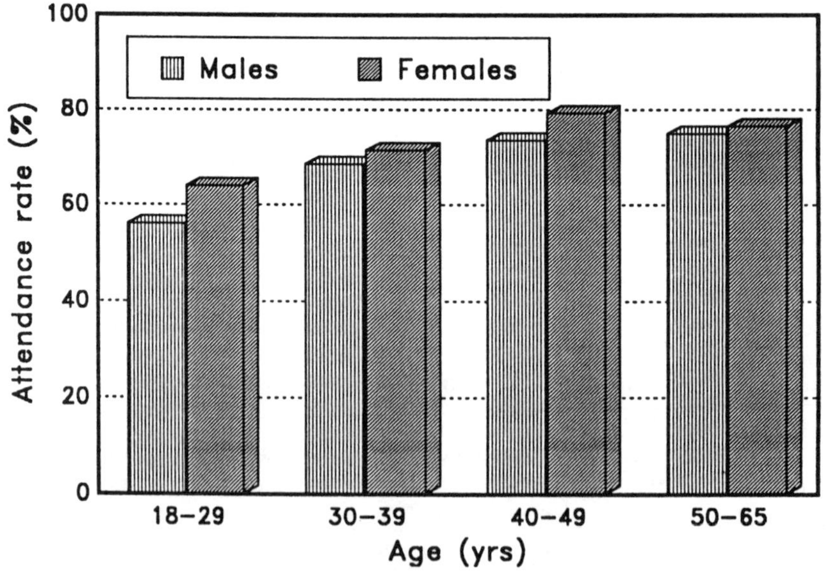

Fig. 1. Attendance by sex and age in 1982 during the prevalence study. (Women vs men: 72.9% vs 68.2%; $X^2 = 7.2$, $P < 0.01$. Increase with age: $X^2_t = 47.7$, $P < 0.001$.)

and 78 (4.1%) had had a previous cholecystectomy for gallstones. Nineteen subjects were excluded from the calculation of prevalence because ultrasonography was not conclusive. The above data refer, therefore, on 1911 subjects. In this number are included 9 persons with biliary sludge, but no gallstones in their gallbladder.

Prevalence was higher in females, and the age standardized Mantel-Haenszel Relative Risk (RR_{MH}) [10] for females was 2.16 (95% c.l. = 1.65 to 2.83) in comparison to males. The prevalence of gallstone disease increased steadily with age in both sexes (Fig. 2).

After 5 yr, in 1987 we reexamined the population of Sirmione with the same protocol, in order to assess the incidence and risk factors of gallstone disease. Besides the 210 subjects with diagnosed gallstone disease, 73 subjects who participated in the first study were either living elsewhere (44) or have died for causes not related to gallstone disease (29). 1325 (81.4%) of the remaining 1628 subjects without gallstone in 1982 participated in the incidence study.

Attendance was similar in both sexes and was slightly higher (P < 0.05) in older age groups (Fig. 3). Therefore, in the Sirmione study the yearly incidence of gallstone disease was 0.6%.

The cumulative 5-yr incidence of gallstone disease was 3%. In fact 33 cases of cholelithiasis and 7 cholecystectomies for gallstones were detected among the population who resulted gallstone-free in 1982.

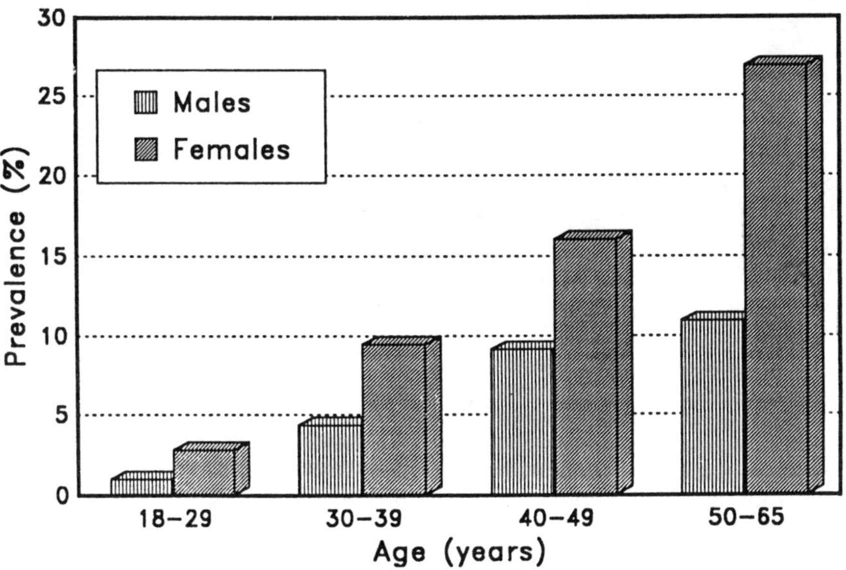

Fig. 2. Prevalence of gallstone disease by sex and age. (Increase with age: males: $X_t^2 = 105.6$, P < 0.001; females: $X_t^2 = 25.4$, P < 0.001).

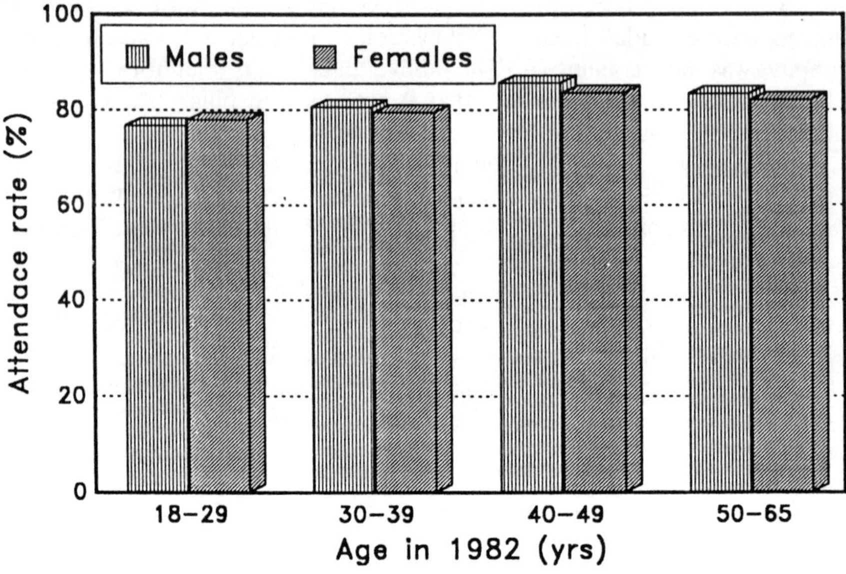

Fig. 3. Attendance by sex and age in 1987 during the incidence study. (Increase with age: X_t^2 = 5.7, P < 0.05).

The incidence rate was higher in the age span 40—65 yr (4.7%) than in youngers subjects (1.2%) (P < 0.001).

Incidence was non-significantly different in males (3.4%) and in females (2.6%).

Conclusion

The Sirmione study has been the first epidemiological study on prevalence and incidence of gallstone disease conducted in a general population sample using ultrasonography for defining cases.

The prevalence study showed that gallstone disease is present in 11% of the adult population. Prevalence is higher in females and increases with ageing.

As far as the incidence study is concerned we confirmed that increasing age is a true risk factor for gallstone development, while we failed to show any sex-related difference. We do not have at the moment any definite explanation for this phenomenon. A more definite answer will possibly derive from the 10-year follow-up study which is planned for 1992.

References

1. Torvik A, Hoivik B (1960): Gallstone in an autopsy series. *Acta Chir Scand* 120: 168—174.
2. Zahor A, Sternby NH, Kagan A, Uemura K, Vanecek R, Vichert AM (1974): Frequency of cholelithiasis in Prague and Malmö: an autopsy study. *Scand J Gastroenterol* 9: 3—7.
3. Holland C, Heaton KH (1972): Increasing frequency of gallbladder operations in the Briston area. *Br Med J* 3: 672—675.
4. Wilbur RS, Bolt RJ (1959): Incidence of gallbladder disease in 'normal' men. *Gastroenterology* 36: 251—255.
5. Gracie WA, Ransohoff DF (1982): The natural history of silent gallstones: the innocent gallstone is not a myth. *N Engl J Med* 307: 798—800.
6. Cooperberg PL, Burhenne HJ (1980): Real time ultrasonography: diagnostic technique of choice in calculous gallbladder disease. *N Engl J Med* 302: 1277—1279.
7. Shapero TF, Rosen IE, Wilson SR (1982): Discrepancy between ultrasound and oral cholecystography in the assessment of gallstone dissolution. *Hepatology* 2: 587—590.
8. Barbara L, Sama C, Morselli Labate AM, Taroni F, Rusticali AG, Festi D, Sapio C, Roda E, Banterle C, Puci A, Formentini F, Colasanti S, Nardin F (1987): A population study on the prevalence of gallstone disease: The Sirmione Study. *Hepatology* 7: 913—917.
9. Barbara L, Festi D, Morselli Labate AM, Rusticali AG, Sama C, Sapio C, Taroni F, Banterle C, Colasanti S, Formentini G, Nardin F, Panzolato G, Puci A, Salvini G (1984): Ultrasonography in the evaluation of the prevalence of gallstone disease: Progetto Sirmione, pp. 73—75 in Labo' G, Bolondi L, Rizzatto G (eds), *Clinical Advances in Ultrasonography* Milano: Masson.
10. Mantel N, Haenszel W (1959): Statistical aspects of the analysis of data from retrospective studies of disease. *J Natl Cancer Inst* 22: 719—748.

3. Gallbladder disease prevalence and cholecystectomy rates

M. C. BATESON

Introduction

The prevalence of gallbladder disease may be measured in various ways, of which autopsy and ultrasonography surveys are most widely used at present. Using them it is possible to compare prevalence in different areas and at different times in the same area.

Critical analysis of rates of surgical treatment for gallbladder disease suggests that there is little relationship to the overall prevalence of disease and that there is also marked variation in rates of surgery over periods of time.

Techniques of assessment

1. *Autopsy survey*

Advantages of this method include the fact that it involves study of existing records and it allows a historical comparison over previous years. Objective evidence is obtained on the presence of common bile duct stones and of cholecystectomy. The appearance of stones can be noted, which is an important clue as to their chemical composition. Large numbers of data can be obtained.

There are certain problems. Most autopsies in Western societies are performed on subjects between the age of 50 and 90 yr and there is less information outside this range. Gallbladder disease rates apparently fluctuate around secular trends, so that it is important to study thousands of autopsies over ten years or more before drawing conclusions. Autopsy rates may vary so that study populations may not be exactly comparable in different years.

The most serious objection to autopsy surveys is that they are not community-based. This does carry the possibility of fallacious conclusions if a condition is associated with other diseases which lead to hospital admission or if it commonly causes death [1]. Neither of these apply to gallbladder

L. Capocaccia et al. (eds), Recent advances in the epidemiology and prevention of gallstone disease, 13—22.

disease, and autopsy prevalence yields valuable information, some of which is not available elsewhere.

2. *Oral cholecystography*

This allows serial or longitudinal study of risk populations such as subjects who have been treated with clofibrate, or had gastric or intestinal surgery. All ages can be studied and information can be obtained about gallstone calcification.

Correlation with symptoms is possible. Problems include a high rate of non-functioning gallbladders, a finding which is difficult to interpret. The procedure depends on patient compliance and absence of pregnancy. Iopanoic acid contrast is not always tolerated well. There is an exposure to ionising radiation. The presence of cholecystectomy can only be determined from the patient's history and presence of compatible scars. The attempt to limit radiation exposure by abbreviated procedures has yielded paradoxical results [2]. One drawback of surveys of populations is that much non-significant gallstone disease is detected, which if revealed to subjects and their doctors may lead to inappropriate cholecystectomy or medical treatment.

3. *Ultrasonography*

This is also suitable for serial and longitudinal studies. All ages and sexes may be easily studied and symptom correlation is possible. Ultrasonography shares many of the disadvantages of oral cholecystectomy surveys. It is not yet a reliable technique for detecting common duct stones and at present there is little past information on ultrasonography prevalence for comparative purposes.

4. *Cholecystectomy rates*

These can discriminate between areas with very low and very high gallstone prevalence, but they do vary a lot independently of gallstone prevalence. Rates have fallen in many countries such as Scotland, the United States, Sweden and Israel, at a time when gallstones remain very common. Women with gallstones seem to come to surgery more frequently than men with gallstones.

5. *Symptoms*

These are often quite misleading in the detection of gallstone disease [3], and at least two-thirds of patients never have any symptoms from their gallstones.

6. *Mortality*

The death rate from gallstone disease is negligible, except for those patients with common bile duct stones, and post-operative deaths in the elderly and frail.

Autopsy gallstone prevalence in dundee

17 058 consecutive Dundee hospital autopsy records from 1953 to May 1989 were analysed, excluding neonatal deaths, since gallstones are very rare before the age of one month. There were adequate details about the gallbladder in 15 311 cases (89.8%).

Gallbladder disease was defined as the presence of gallstones or gravel in the gallbladder or bile ducts; or a surgically removed gallbladder, which usually implies previous symptomatic gallstone disease.

Data were standardised for age and sex. It was noted that there was marked year-to-year fluctuation, and even when figures were grouped into three-year periods this was not completely compensated (Figs. 1, 2). The explanation of this fluctuation is not clear [4]. It may be a true biological effect, but means that great caution must be exercised before drawing conclusions about short-term changes in gallbladder disease prevalence. It is unknown whether such fluctuations will also affect ultrasonography surveys.

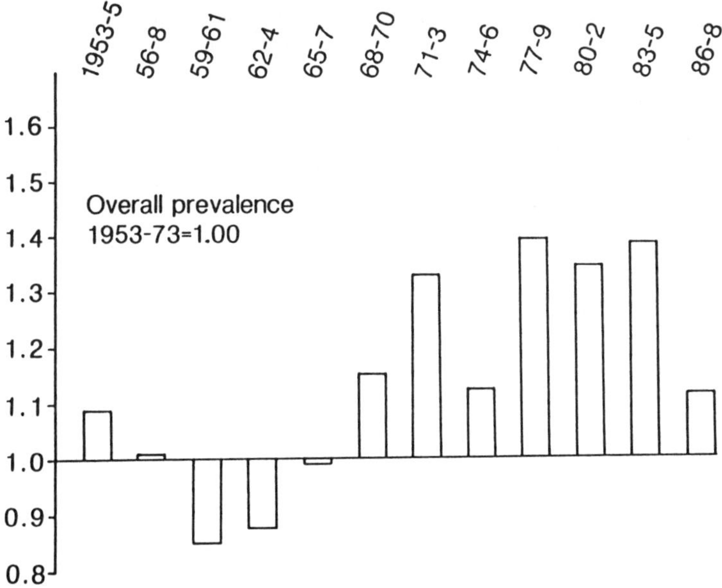

Fig. 1. Standardised prevalence gallbladder disease for women 1953—88.

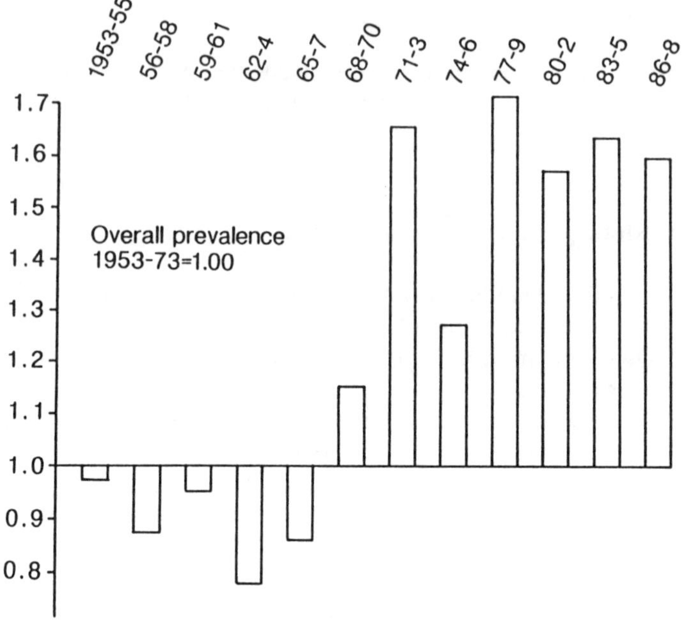

Fig. 2. Standardised prevalence gallbladder disease for men 1953—88.

The analysis of standardised three-year prevalence figures indicates that in the 1970's and 1980's there was more gallbladder disease than had previously been seen in the 1950's and 60's, and this applies to both sexes and all ages (Figs. 3—6). There is a small amount of information from the years 1902—09 and 1936—38 in Dundee, when standardised gallbladder disease prevalence appeared the same as in 1953—73. The figures for 1953—73 are similar also to standardised autopsy prevalence of gallbladder disease in 9351 autopsies in Leeds 1910—26 [5], and 13 115 in Leeds 1930—49 [6].

It may be concluded that the prevalence of gallbladder disease in hospital autopsies was the same for England and Scotland in the past, but for Scotland at least there has been a true increase in gallbladder disease prevalence in the last 20 yr.

During the analysis of autopsy data it became clear that there has been a recent fall in the number of autopsies performed in Dundee, even though the hospital departments and catchment population have not changed significantly. From 1953—73 there were 500—650 autopsies annually. The figure peaked in 1976 when there were 693 autopsies, but the figure has continuously declined since then to 260 autopsies in 1987 and 244 autopsies in 1988 (Fig. 7).

The reason for this fall, which has been documented in other centres also, is a lower rate of autopsies requested by clinicians, possibly reflecting a mistaken confidence in the ability to diagnose conditions completely before

GALLSTONE PREVALENCE 1974–89 & 1953–73

AGE	0-9	10-39	40-49	50-59	60-69	70-79	80-89	90+
Women 1974-89	0/30	5/72	11/76	66/250	190/609	330/1001	383/895	63/138
1953-73	0/184	10/201	30/249	90/569	272/1069	380/1317	233/755	23/65
Men 1974-89	0/19	6/83	6/103	36/330	112/704	255/1094	128/487	24/56
1953-73	0/243	4/261	15/342	50/802	142/1434	191/1259	102/569	11/45

Fig. 3. Numbers with gallbladder disease 1953—89.

GALLSTONE PREVALENCE 1974–89 & 1953–73

AGE	0-9	10-39	40-49	50-59	60-69	70-79	80-89	90+
Women 1974-89	.	6.9%	14.5%	26.4%	31.2%	33%	42.8%	45.7%
1953-73	.	5.0%	12%	15.8% ***	25.4% ***	28.9% ***	30.9% ***	35.4%
Men 1974-89	.	7.2%	5.8%	10.9%	15.9%	23.3%	26.2%	42.9%
1953-73	.	1.5%	4.4%	6.2% **	9.9% ***	15.2% ***	17.9% **	24.4%

** p < .01
*** p < .001

Fig. 4. Percentages with gallbladder disease 1953—89.

death. The fall in hospital autopsy rates has serious implications for effective medical audit.

World-wide prevalence of gallbladder disease

There is only a small amount of information comparing the results of cholecystography, ultrasonography and autopsy studies in the same populations, but such data as there are suggests that the results are similar. It is, therefore, possible to set up a world league table of gallbladder disease prevalence (Fig. 8). Generally African and black populations have a lower prevalence whereas North American, European, South African and Antipodean whites have a high rate, and North American Indians and their descendants have the highest rate of all.

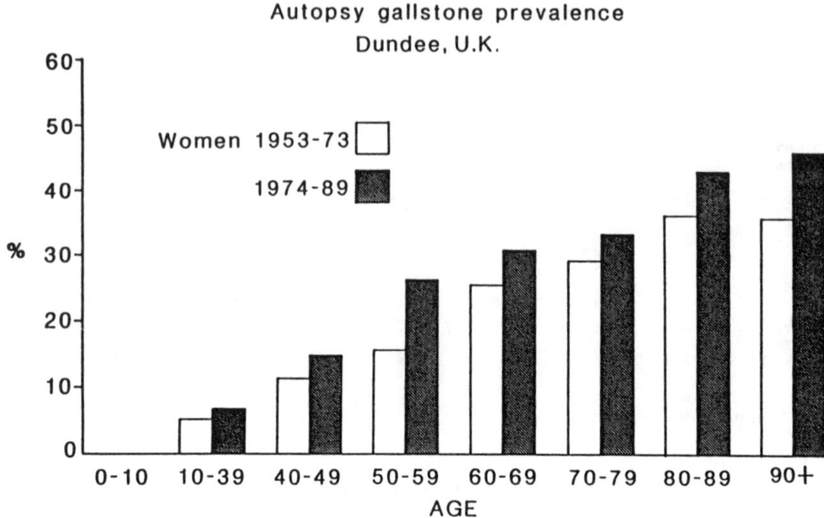

Fig. 5. Proportions of women with gallbladder disease 1953—89.

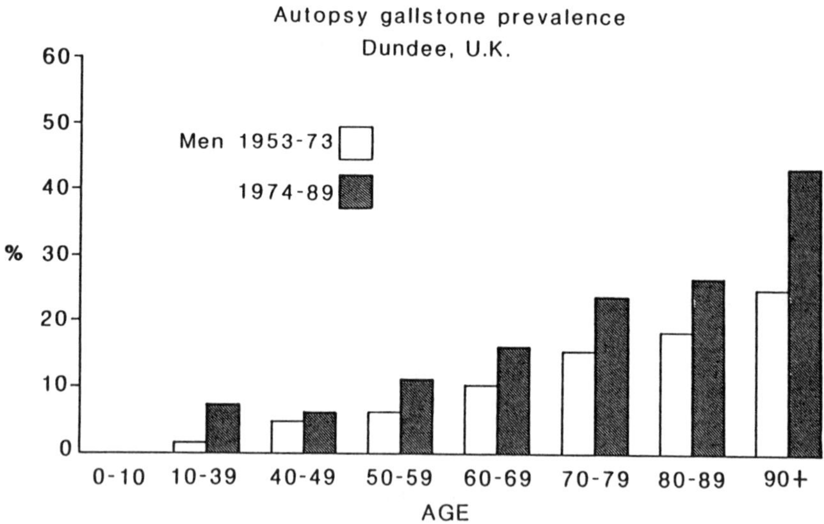

Fig. 6. Proportions of men with gallbladder disease 1953—89.

The data are patchy from Africa and Asia. It is not clear how far differences are explained by race rather than environment, but it would not be difficult to collect further information about this. For instance, ultrasonography surveys of Japanese in Japan and second generation Japanese in other

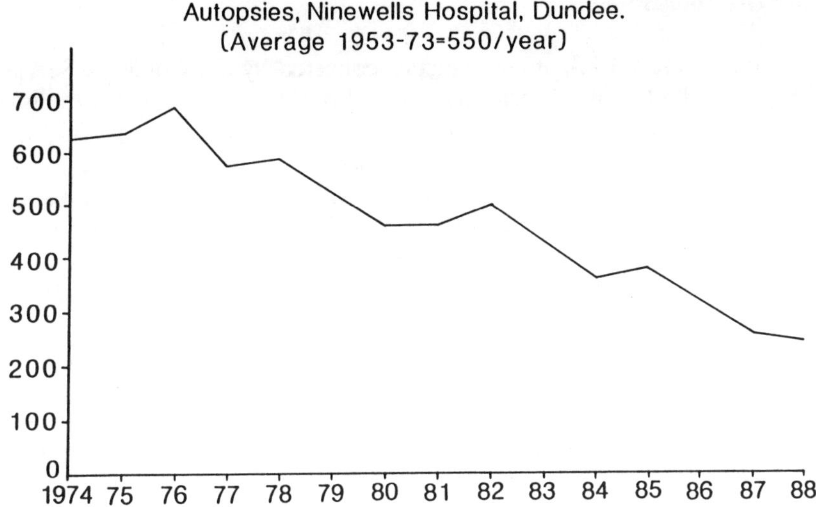

Fig. 7. Decline in number of autopsies 1974—88.

WORLD RECORD	VERY HIGH	HIGH	MODERATE	LOW
North American Indians	USA Mexican Americans	USA Whites	USA Blacks	RSA Blacks
		Panama Whites	Panama Blacks	Egypt
Pima	Chile	USA Puerto Ricans	Japan	Zambia
Chippewa	Sweden	RSA Whites	Singapore Chinese	Nigeria
MicMac	Czechoslovakia	Australia	Greece	
Sioux		Great Britain	Ireland	
Navajo		Italy	Romania	
		Denmark		
		West Germany		
		Norway		
		Holland		
		Kashmir		

NB:　USA = United States of America

　　　RSA = Republic of South Africa

Fig. 8. Worldwide prevalence of gallbladder disease.

countries would yield valuable information about the role of diet. The American Indians are considered to be the same ethnic stock as the Eskimos, whose natural diet is quite different. It would be very intriguing to study Eskimos to see if they experience the same high gallbladder disease prevalence.

Cholecystectomy rates

The Scottish hospital in-patient statistics collected by the Common Services Agency record all cholecystectomies carried out in Scotland under the NHS since 1961. This provides data on more than 90% of such surgery since there has been little tradition of private medicine in this country.

The population of Scotland has been steady at around 5.2 million until 1981, but fell slightly to 5.1 million in 1987. Data were analysed by age and sex for all Scotland (Fig. 9). Total numbers of cholecystectomies in the Dundee hospitals were analysed separately and showed similar trends (Fig. 10).

There were very few operations in patients under 10 yr or over 90 yr, but otherwise from 1961—77 there was a continuous rise in the number of operations which was then followed by a sharp fall. There was fluctuation in the years 1982—83 reflecting industrial unrest in the health service and a subsequent catch-up period.

For all Scotland there were 2438 cholecystectomies in 1961, 5722 in 1977 and 4511 in 1988. For the city of Dundee the figures were 71 in 1961, 320 in 1978 and 213 in 1988. An increasing proportion of operations was in the age group 70—89 (for men 10.7% in 1961, 22.5% in 1987; for women 9.8% in 1961, 15.9% in 1987). There was also a very marked rise in the proportion of cholecystectomies which were performed in women aged 10—39, from 16.6% in 1961 to 24.7% in 1971, and 27% in 1987 (Fig. 11). This was not seen for men aged 10—39 (9.8% in 1961 and 10.7% in 1987).

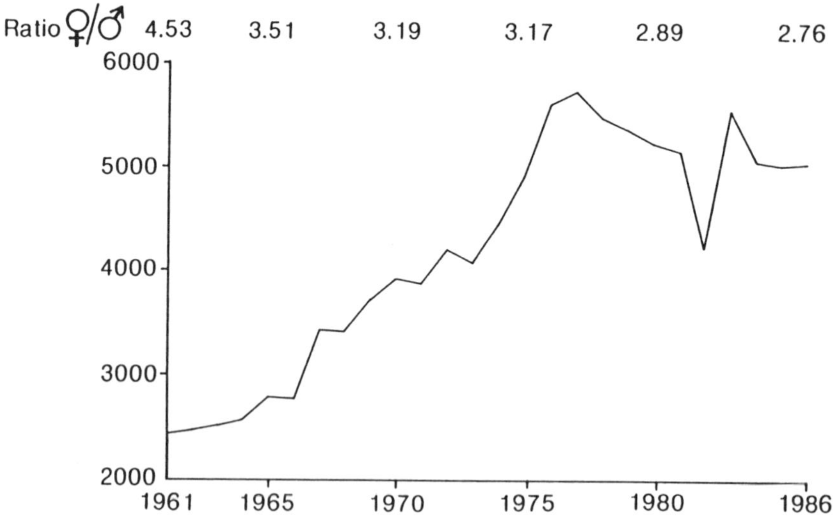

Fig. 9. Numbers of cholecystectomies in Scotland performed under the National Health Service, figures from Scottish Hospital In-patient Statistics.

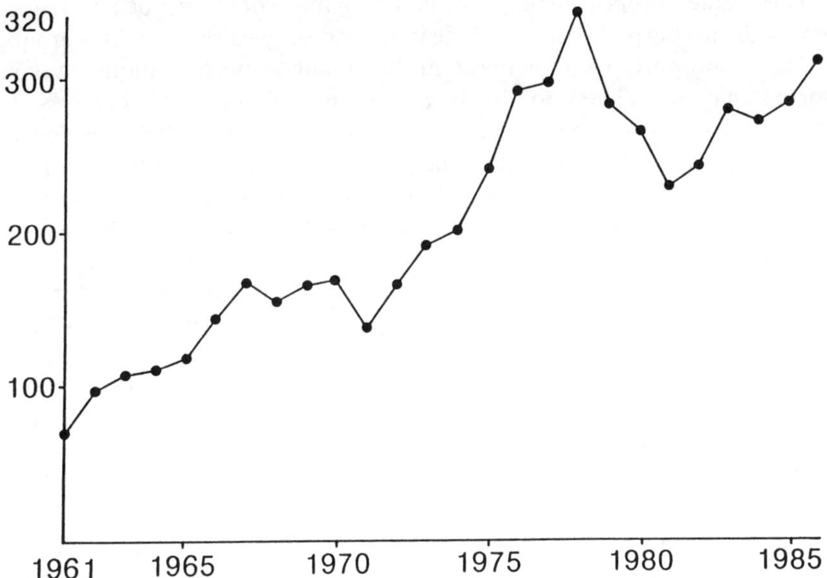

Fig. 10. Numbers of cholecystectomies in Dundee, NHS figures from Scottish Hospital in-patient statistics.

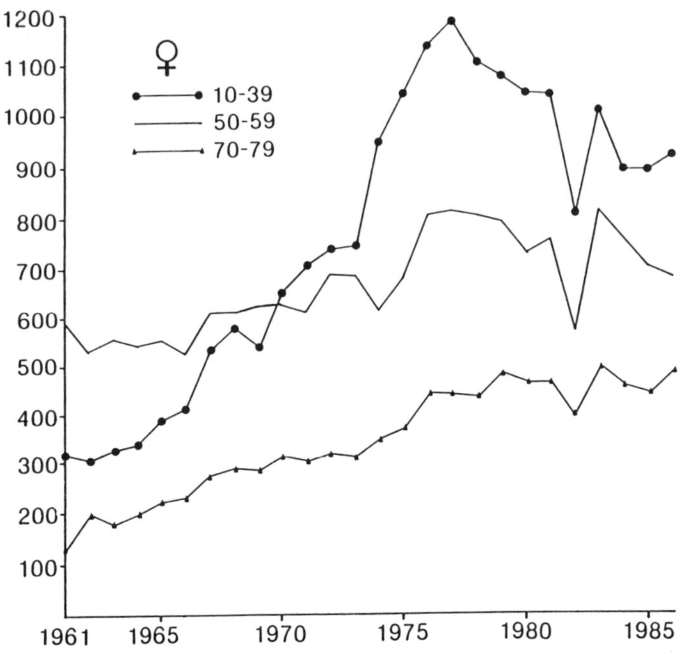

Fig. 11. Change in numbers of cholecystectomies in Scottish women of different ages.

The greater proportion of operations in the elderly is not surprising in view of the ageing population and the improved surgical results in this group.

The disproportionate increase in the number of operations in young women may be related to the increased use of oral contraceptives, first introduced in 1959. These agents do not appear to alter the prevalence of gallstones, but they may accelerate the performance of cholecystectomy [7].

In the years 1974—89 in the Dundee autopsy survey 17.6% of women with gallbladder disease had had a cholecystectomy and 11.8% of men. Though it is not disputed that men are different from women, this particular difference did not achieve statistical significance! Overall about one in seven of these patients had come to surgery, which compares with a similar cholecystectomy rate in gallstone disease in Spain, but is much lower than in Italy and the United States of America where about one in three subjects with gallstones have had a cholecystectomy. This difference probably relates more to surgical practice than any true difference in gallstone disease.

These figures show that there is a poor correlation between gallstone disease prevalence and cholecystectomy rates. The fall in surgical activity rates since the late 1970's may reflect a better understanding of the harmlessness of many gallstones and the development of alternative methods of treatment. It has been seen also in Sweden, in Israel, and in the U.S.A., where an 18% fall in the numbers of cholecystectomies was seen between 1980—86.

References

1.   Mainland D (1953): The risk of fallacious conclusions from autopsy data on the incidence of diseases with applications to heart disease. *American Heart Journal* 45: 644—654.
2.   Bainton D, Davies GT, Evans KT, Gravelle IH (1976): Gallbladder disease: Prevalence in a South Wales industrial town. *New England Journal of Medicine* 294: 1147—1149.
3.   Glambek I, Arnesio B, Soreide O (1989): Correlation between gallstones and abdominal symptoms in a random population. *Scandinavian Journal of Gastroenterology* 24: 277—281.
4.   Balzer K, Goebell H, Breuer N, Ruping KW, Leder LD (1986): Epidemiology of gallstones in a German industrial town (Essen) from 1940—1975. *Digestion* 33: 189—197.
5.   Gross D (1929): A statistical study of cholelithiasis. *Journal of Pathology and Bacteriology* 32: 503—526.
6.   Watkinson G (1967): The autopsy incidence of gallstones in England and Scotland. *Proceedings Third World Congress of Gastroenterology, Tokyo* 4: 125—130.
7.   Royal College of General Practitioners' Oral Contraception Study (1982): Oral contraceptives and gallbladder disease. *Lancet* 2: 957—959.

4. Prevalence of clinical gallbladder disease in Mexican Americans

A. K. DIEHL

Hispanic Americans now consititute the second largest minority group in the United States, after blacks. Heavy immigration and high birth rates have resulted in their rapid growth in numbers and importance in American society over the past several decades. The term 'Hispanic' as used in the United States today encompasses several ethnic subgroups. Mexican Americans, Cuban Americans, Spanish Americans, Puerto Ricans, and other Hispanic populations may share a common language, but they differ in their history, culture, and genetic heritage. It is important for epidemiologic studies to discriminate among the various Hispanic American groups [1].

Mexican Americans represent the largest Hispanic subpopulation in the United States. The 1980 national census counted 8.7 million Spanish-surnamed persons of Mexican origin, or 3.9% of the population. Mexican Americans are concentrated in five southwestern states (Texas, Colorado, New Mexico, Arizona, and California), but large numbers also live in Chicago and other major cities. Ethnically, Mexican Americans are the descendants of marriages between pre-Columbian native peoples (Amerindians) and European immigrants, beginning with the Spanish conquistadors. Over the centuries, these populations have merged to create a 'mestizo' (mixed) society which differs genetically and culturally from other North American groups. Recent studies of Mexican Americans in Texas have found that 15 to 45% of their genetic markers are of Amerindian origin [2—4].

Physicians practicing in areas with large concentrations of Mexican Americans have long been impressed by the seemingly high rates and early age at onset of gallstone disease in this population group. Case series describing cholecystectomies done in adolescents in San Antonio, Texas have remarked on the preponderance of Mexican American patients. Similarly, reports from California have commented on the high rates of gallstone disease in Mexican Americans. Additional studies have documented a high mortality due to gallbladder cancer in persons of Mexican origin. Since this cancer is closely associated with the presence of gallstones, its incidence is believed to reflect gallstone prevalence in the population. Despite these

L. Capocaccia et al. (eds), Recent advances in the epidemiology and prevention of gallstone disease, 23—28.
© 1991 *Kluwer Academic Publishers. Printed in the Netherlands.*

reports, few quantitative data on the prevalence of gallbladder disease in Mexican Americans were available until recently [2].

Prompted by these reports and our observations as clinicians, we performed a cross-sectional analysis of medical records from the Family Health Center of the University of Texas Health Science Center at San Antonio. Study subjects were low-income women enrolled with their families in a special program which offered comprehensive health care without charge. All subjects completed a detailed medical history on enrollment in the Family Health Center. From the 3389 women aged 15 to 59 who had entered the practice, we selected all 356 blacks, 111 non-Hispanic whites, and an age-stratified random sample of Mexican Americans to create a final study population of 1018 women. 'Clinical gallbladder disease' was defined as a hospital record of surgery for gallstones, a subject report of past cholecystectomy, or a record of an abnormal oral cholecystogram (stones or non-visualization). Medical records were reviewed to determine age- and ethnic group-specific prevalences of clinical gallbladder disease.

Our results confirmed our clinical suspicion of high rates of gallbladder disease among Mexican Americans. Mexican American prevalences were higher than those of non-Hispanic whites and blacks for each age stratum. The age-standardized rates for women ages 15 to 59 were 14.4% for Mexican Americans, 9.2% for non-Hispanic whites, and 4.7% for blacks. In a log-linear model analysis, these ethnic differences remained significant ($p < 0.001$) after age, relative weight, and diabetes mellitus were taken into account [5]. We further compared the prevalences found in this study with those determined by the same methodology in the Pima Indian women of southern Arizona and in the women of Framingham, Massachusetts [6, 7]. Clinical gallbladder disease prevalence in San Antonio Mexican Americans ages 30—59 was lower than that of Pima Indians, but considerably higher than that of non-Hispanic whites in Framingham (Fig. 1). We hypothesized that the elevated prevalence in Mexican American women might be related to their Amerindian genetic heritage [5].

Subsequent to this initial report, we have performed a series of epidemiological studies on clinical gallbladder disease using data collected during the San Antonio Heart Study. The San Antonio Heart Study is a population-based health survey performed between October 1979 and November 1982. Its primary purpose is to assess the prevalence of cardiovascular risk factors and diabetes in a bicultural sample of Mexican Americans and 'Anglo' Americans (non-Hispanic whites) in San Antonio, Texas. Subjects from 25 to 64 yr of age were randomly selected from three neighborhoods: two low-income census tracts in an almost exclusively Mexican American section of the city ('barrio') where a highly traditional Mexican American cultural orientation has been maintained; two middle-income ('transitional') census tracts which have approximately equal numbers of Mexican Americans and non-Hispanic whites; and a cluster of high income census tracts ('suburbs') which is about 90% non-Hispanic white and 10% Mexican American. Only

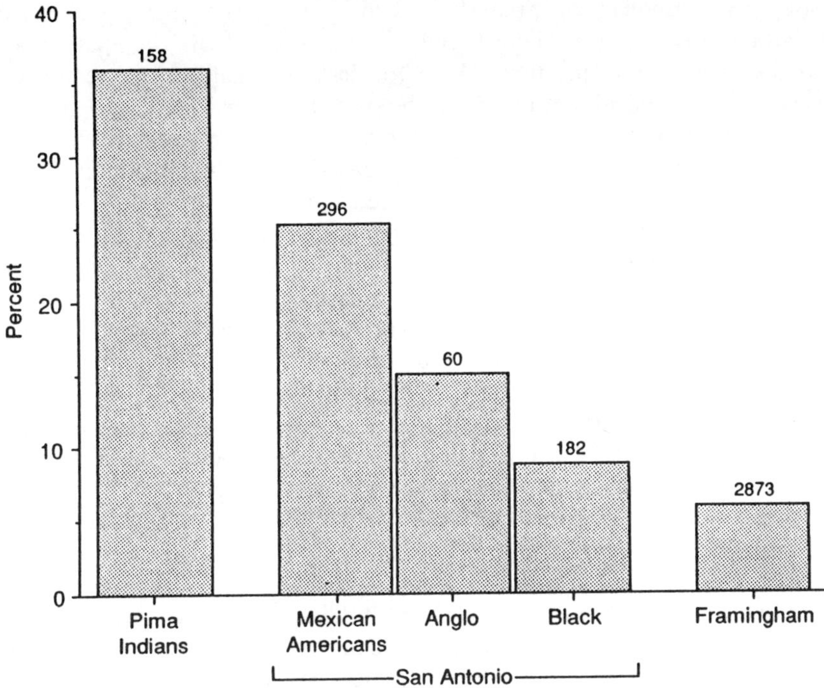

Fig. 1. Prevalence of clinical gallbladder disease in women ages 30—59: Pima Indians; Mexican Americans, non-Hispanic whites (Anglos), and blacks in San Antonio; and non-Hispanic whites in Framingham, Massachusetts. Data from references [5—7].

Mexican Americans were sampled in the barrio, and approximately equal numbers of each ethnic group were sampled in the transitional and suburban neighborhoods, where stratified random sampling was performed. Subjects' ethnic classification was based on Spanish or non-Spanish surname of both parents (maiden name in the case of the mother), birthplace of parents, participant's preferred ethnic identity, and stated ethnicity of all four grandparents. Offspring of interethnic marriages, Hispanics of non-Mexican heritage, and Orientals were excluded from these analyses.

The study consisted of a home interview followed by a medical examination in a mobile clinic. Response rates to the home interviews ranged from 85.3% in the transitional neighborhood to 89.0% in the barrio. Of those interviewed, 97% were deemed eligible for the medical exam; reasons for exclusion included moving out of the area and the discovery of pregnancy after the interview. Response rates to the medical exam ranged from 68.9% in the barrio to 80.4% in the suburbs.

The home interview was extensive and covered a wide range of demographic, nutritional, sociological, and attitudinal items. The presence of clinical gallbladder disease was determined from the home interview. The interviewer asked each participant three questions relating to gallbladder disease, using English or Spanish according to participant's preference. Gallbladder disease was considered to be present if the participant responded 'yes' to the question, 'Have you had your gallbladder removed?' Disease was also considered present if the participant answered 'yes' to 'Have you ever had an X-ray taken of your gallbladder?', and in addition answered 'stones' to 'What did the doctor say the X-ray showed?' Gallbladder disease was considered absent if the patient denied cholecystectomy and reported never having had cholecystography, or reported previous cholecystography with normal findings. A small number of participants who had undergone cholecystography with equivocal findings and had not had gallbladder surgery were considered to have uncertain status, and were not included in the analysis. Although the determination of clinical gallbladder disease from subjects' histories may occasionally be in error, Bernstein et al. have found this method to be valid when compared to physicians' records. Using the question, 'Has a doctor ever told you that you had gallbladder disease'?, they estimated 97% simple agreement between subject responses and physician reports [8]. Nevertheless, this method understimates the true prevalence of cholelithiasis, as persons unaware of undiagnosed 'silent' stones are not counted.

Our final study population consisted of 2990 subjects, of whom 60% were Mexican American and 40% were non-Hispanic white. Fifty-six percent were women. As expected, the prevalence of clinical gallbladder disease increased with age and was greater in women than in men. Prevalences were consistently greater in Mexican American women than in non-Hispanic white women (Fig. 2). In men, differences between the two ethnic groups were small. In Mexican American women, gallbladder disease prevalence rose from 8.3% for ages 25—34 years to 27.7% for ages 55—64 years. In non-Hispanic white women, prevalence ranged from 5.5% in those 25—34 yr to 16.7% in those 55—64 yr. The age-standardized prevalence in Mexican American women was 16.9% versus 8.7% in non-Hispanic whites (p < 0.0001). In men fewer cases were observed. The age-standardized prevalence in Mexican American men was 4.2% versus 3.4% in non-Hispanic whites (not significant) [9].

We further explored these ethnic differences in a series of stratified analyses. The study population was grouped by levels of body mass index (3 strata), parity (4 strata), neighborhood of residence (3 strata), educational attainment (4 strata), occupational status (3 strata), and family income (3 strata). Age- and sex-standardized prevalences of clinical gallbladder disease were calculated for Mexican Americans and non-Hispanic whites in each stratum. In 17 of 19 comparisons, the prevalences were higher in Mexican Americans [9]. Recent publications from the San Antonio Heart study have demonstrated that the higher prevalence of clinical gallbladder disease in Mexican Americans persists after adjustment for age, body mass index, body fat distribution, nutrient intake (assessed by 24 hour diet recall), and diabetes mellitus during multiple logistic regression analyses. In general, ethnic differ-

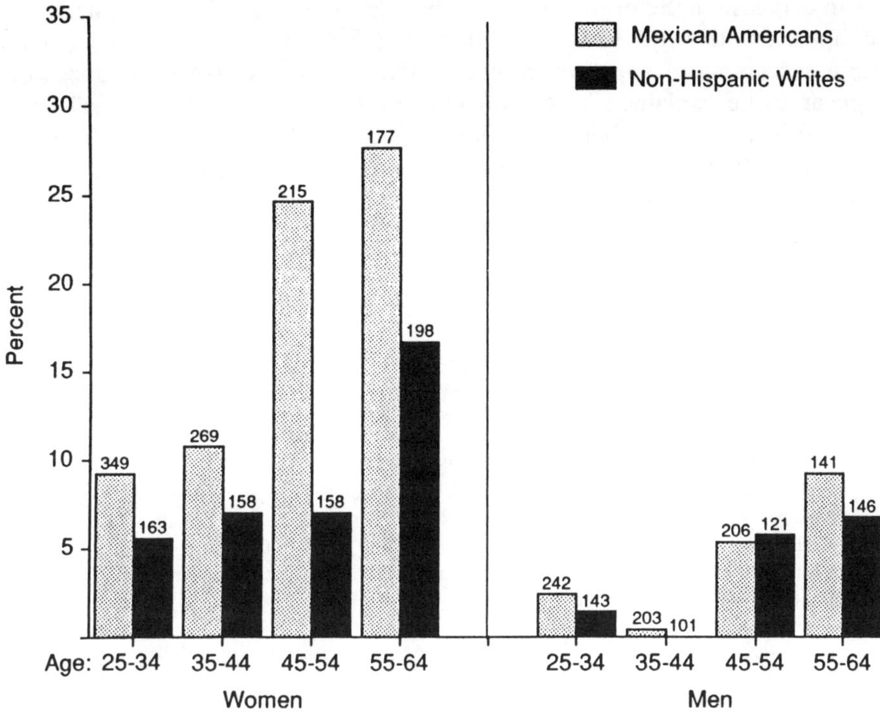

Fig. 2. Prevalence of clinical gallbladder disease in Mexican Americans and non-Hispanic whites in the San Antonio Heart Study. Data from reference [9].

ences are more pronounced in women, and the estimated odds ratios for gallbladder disease range between 1.5 and 2 times those of non-Hispanic whites [10–12].

Since 1985, the increased risk of gallbladder disease in Mexican Americans has been confirmed by three additional reports. Hanis et al. reported the prevalence of clinical gallbladder disease (history of 'gallbladder trouble' or a 'gallbladder operation') among the Mexican American population of Starr County, Texas [13]. They found that Mexican Americans have a prevalence of cholecystectomy twice that of the Framingham population. Arevalo et al. reviewed autopsy records in San Francisco and found that 'Latino' women have a prevalence of gallstones twice that of non-Hispanic whites [14]. Maurer et al. reported population-based prevalences of cholelithiasis determined by ultrasonography in Mexican Americans, Cuban Americans, and Puerto Ricans participating in the Hispanic Health and Nutrition Examination Survey. They found age-adjusted prevalences of gallstone disease in Mexican Americans to be 1.5 to 1.8 times those of the other two Hispanic groups [15]. Finally, Samet et al. surveyed a Spanish American community near Albuquerque, New Mexico and found rates of previous cholecystectomy similar to those observed in the Starr County Mexican Americans [13, 16].

In conclusion, the prevalence of gallbladder disease in Mexican Americans is approximately 1.5 to 2 times that of non-Hispanic whites. The ethnic difference is more apparent in women than in men. However, it does not appear to be explained by confounding by other risk factors for gallstone disease including age, body mass index, body fat distribution, parity, socio-economic status, diet, or diabetes mellitus. The possible genetic basis of this ethnic difference will be discussed in Chapter 13.

References

1. Diehl AK (1988): The melting pot: examine before stirring. *J Gen Int Med* 3: 90—91.
2. Diehl AK, Stern MP (1989): Special health problems of Mexican Americans: obesity, gallbladder disease, diabetes mellitus, and cardiovascular disease. *Adv Intern Med* 34: 73—96.
3. Hanis CL, Chakraborty R, Ferrell RE, Schull WJ (1986): Individual admixture estimates: disease associations and individual risk of diabetes and gallbladder disease among Mexican Americans in Starr County, Texas. *Am J Phys Anthropol* 70: 433—444.
4. Chakraborty R, Ferrell RE, Stern MP et al. (1986): Relationship of prevalence of non-insulin dependent diabetes mellitus to Amerindian admixture in the Mexican Americans of San Antonio, Texas. *Genet Epidemiol* 3: 435—454.
5. Diehl AK, Stern MP, Ostrower VS, Friedman PC (1980): Prevalence of clinical gallbladder disease in Mexican American, Anglo, and black women. *South Med J* 73: 438—441, 443.
6. Comess LJ, Bennett PH, Burch TA (1967): Clinical gallbladder disease in Pima Indians: its high prevalence in contrast to Framingham, Massachusetts. *N Engl J Med* 277: 894—898.
7. Friedman GD, Kannel WB, Dawber TR (1966): The epidemiology of gallbladder disease: observations in the Framingham study. *J Chron Dis* 19: 273—292.
8. Bernstein RA, Giefer EE, Rimm AA (1976): Gallbladder disease. I. Assessment of validity and reliability of data derived from a questionnaire. *J Chron Dis* 29: 51—58.
9. Diehl AK, Rosenthal M, Hazuda HP, Comeaux PJ, Stern MP (1985): Socioeconomic status and the prevalence of clinical gallbladder disease. *J Chron Dis* 38: 1019—1026.
10. Haffner SM, Diehl AK, Stern MP, Hazuda HP (1989): Central adiposity and gallbladder disease in Mexican Americans. *Am J Epidemiol* 129: 587—595.
11. Diehl AK, Haffner SM, Knapp JA, Hazuda HP, Stern, MP (1989): Dietary intake and the prevalence of gallbladder disease in Mexican Americans. *Gastroenterology* 97: 1527—1533.
12. Haffner SM, Diehl AK, Mitchell BD, Stern MP, Hazuda HP (1990): Increased prevalence of clinical gallbaldder disease in subjects with non-insulin dependent diabetes mellitus. *Am J Epidemiol* 132: 327—335.
13. Hanis CL, Ferrell RE, Tulloch BR, Schull WJ (1985): Gallbladder disease epidemiology in Mexican Americans in Starr County, Texas. *Am J Epidemiol* 122: 820—829.
14. Arevalo JA, Wollitzer AO, Corporon MB, Larios M, Huante D, Ortiz MT (1987): Ethnic variability in cholelithiasis — an autopsy study. *West J Med* 147: 44—47.
15. Maurer KR, Everhart JE, Ezzati TM, Johannes RS, Knowler WC, Larson DL, Sanders R, Shawker TH, Roth HP (1989): Prevalence of gallstone disease in Hispanic populations in the United States. *Gastroenterology* 96: 487—492.
16. Samet JM, Coultas, DB, Howard CA, Skipper BJ, Hanis CL (1988): Diabetes, gallbladder disease, obesity, and hypertension among Hispanics in New Mexico. *Am J Epidemiol* 128: 1302—1311.

5. The Italian multicenter study on epidemiology and prevention of cholelithiasis (MICOL): ultrasonographic standardization

D. FESTI, L. LALLONI, F. TARONI, L. BARBARA, A. MENOTTI, G. RICCI and THE MICOL GROUP*

Introduction

The Italian multicenter study on Epidemiology and Prevention of Gallstone Disease (MICOL), which is currently under way in 18 centres on a study population of about 60 000 subjects, adopted Ultrasonography (U.S.) as the detection tool for stones in the gallbladder.

The choice was dictated by the higher performance of U.S. in the diagnosis of gallstones as compared to cholecystography [1—3], and by its safety and efficacy in the study of large population groups, as recently shown by two epidemiologic studies already performed in Italy [4—6].

Since several ultrasonographers were to be involved, a study to assess U.S. reliability in the diagnosis of gallstones, under uniform and controlled conditions, was performed before starting the field study, in order to asses the degree of agreement of trained ultrasonographers using fixed criteria of interpretation and recommended imaging techniques.

Because a 'true' diagnosis as to the presence of gallstones was not available, the appraisal was focused on the issues of inter and intraobserver variability. Divergence in applying the agreed criteria was tested by having the same U.S. image interpreted by all the observers (interobserver variability), while inconsistency in their use by the same observer was investigated by asking each of them to rate twice the same image (intraobserver variability).

The purpose of the reliability study was twofold:
1. to measure the level of agreement between observers and within each of them in order to ascertain whether they needed further training;
2. to identify the most often misclassified images and the most usual types of misclassification in order to revise and/or sharpen diagnostic criteria.

---

* For the composition of the MICOL group see p. xi (list of contributors).

L. Capocaccia et al. (eds), Recent advances in the epidemiology and prevention of gallstone disease, 29—35.
© 1991 *Kluwer Academic Publishers. Printed in the Netherlands.*

Methods

Trainees and training program

Fortysix observers from 18 centres were chosen as trainees; all of them had been using U.S. for at least 6 months, (17 for < 1 yr, 10 for 1 to 3 yr and for 19 > 3 yr).

Nine were radiologists, 17 were practicing in departments of internal medicine and 20 in departments of gastroenterology. All of them attended the whole training program and followed the reliability study. The first step of the training program was a one-day workshop, chaired by two of the authors (D.F. and L.L.), designed to establish precise criteria for both U.S. techniques and the diagnosis of gallstones.

Since all the participating centres had the same type of real-time ecographer equipped with a 3.5 MHz. linear transducer, the decision was taken to examine the subjects after an overnight fast in 3 consecutive standard positions (supine, left lateral and standing), in order to confirm the presence of gallstones and to evaluate the mobility of gallstone-related U.S. images in subsequent scans.

After an extensive review of the available studies [1—3, 7], the following U.S. images were accepted as criteria for the diagnosis of stones in the gallbladder:

1. one (or more) echogenic, distally shadowing possibly movable structures within the gallbladder;
2. non-shadowing echoes within the gallbladder;
3. echogenic structures with constant shadowing in the region of the gallbladder fossa, with no or poor visualization of the gallbladder.

The visualization of multiple weak echoes in the dependent portion of the gallbladder, with no accompanying acoustic shadow and slow changes in the fluid-fluid level as the decubitus modifies, was accepted as suggestive of biliary sludge.

Diagnostic criteria and examination rules were exhaustively illustrated in a booklet, which was sent to the trainees.

Furthermore, a one-week training period in the two leading U.S. centres was offered to all the echographers to make them well acquainted with the equipment and the agreed criteria.

Procedures in the reading of U.S. images

During a two-day meeting, the 46 ultrasonographers were asked to read U.S. images of the gallbladder recorded on a videotape film. Test images were recorded during routine U.S. examinations of the gallbladder of 50 out-patients from two participating centres using the same equipment available for the field study.

Case histories were selected in order to offer the whole spectrum of images most likely to occur. The 90 min film included 58 images, 8 of which were duplicated and inserted twice in order to evaluate intraobserver variability.

The observers, unaware of case histories, were asked to read the film in a wide, quiet room where ten booths had been prepared, each provided with a videotape. They were allowed to examine each image as long as they wanted, 1hr being the overall examination time.

The observers were asked to classify images as 'Inconclusive' or 'Doubtful' when the poor quality of U.S. images or their own uncertainty prevented conclusive evidence, and as 'Definite' in the presence or absence of gallstones and sludge, according to the agreed criteria. Futhermore, positive cases were rated for the number of gallstones (single, multiple or unassessable).

Statistical analysis

The extent of agreement between and within the 46 observers was assessed using the proportion of overall agreement and the unweighed Kappa-statistics [8—9]. Overall proportions of agreement between the 46 observers on each of the 50 cases were evaluated in order to identify the most often misinterpreted U.S. images. Since this statistics does not adjust for the agreement expected by chance alone, the extent of agreement beyond chance between the 46 observers on rating all the 50 cases, and within each observer on rating twice the same 8 cases, was assessed by means of the Kappa statistics.

The Kappa statistics can be interpreted as an estimate of the probability of agreement between two randomly selected observers on rating a randomly selected case, adjusted for the agreement expected by chance,

The general form of the K-coefficient is

$$K = \frac{Po - pc}{1 - pc},$$

where Po is the proportion of the observed agreement and pc is the proportion of agreement expected by chance. Fleiss' generalization of the Kappa statistics was adopted to assess agreement across categories (Overall Kappa) and on each nominal category (Category Specific Kappa Statistics), where both the categories and the observers are more than 2 and the number of ratings per case is constant and equal to the total number of observers (i.e. each observer rates each case) [8].

Interobservers variability in rating the presence of gallstones was estimated by means of the Landis and Koch's extension of the Kappa statistics to the case of > 2 cases rated into $K = 2$ categories when the number of observers is unequal for each case [10].

The scores of the Kappa statistics can vary from $+ 1$ (perfect agreement) to 0 (observed agreement equal to agreement expected by chance) to negative values (down to -1) when the observed agreement is lower than the agreement expected by chance.

Fleiss [8] proposed that the observed proportion of agreement beyond chance be rated 'excellent' for Kappa values $\geqslant 0.75$ and 'poor' for values $\leqslant 0.40$, whereas values between 0.40 and 0.74 represent 'fair' (0.41 to 0.59) or 'good' (0.60 to 0.74) agreement respectively. Although these cut-off points are widely arbitrary and closer limits for Kappa scores have been proposed [10], they can provide useful tools to evaluate the results.

Additionally, types of disagreement were explored comparing the Modal Frequency Category of each case (i.e. the category in which the largest proportion of observers rated each case) with its second most frequent category.

Results

The proportion of overall agreement between observers for the four main diagnostic categories of the study (Gallstone; No Gallstone; Doubtful Examination; Inconclusive Examination) reached 90% in 33 cases and 50—90% in 16; in 1 case only the overall agreement was $< 50\%$.

The scores of the overall and category specific Kappa statistics for inter-observer agreement suggest 'good' agreement for the four main diagnostic categories (K overall $= 0.649$) and for the 'No Gallstone' category ($K = 0.725$), while 'excellent' agreement ($K = 0.784$) exists for the 'Gallstone' category.

The very poor agreement on rating examinations as 'Doubtful' or 'Inconclusive' ($K = 0.137$ and $K = 0.115$ respectively) suggests that these categories were widely used to overcome observers' uncertanties.

The relation between the experience in abdominal U.S. and the observed agreement was investigated comparing the overall and category specific Kappa scores observed in two selected groups of observers, i.e. observers with < 1 yr ('novices') and > 3 yr experience in abdominal U.S. ('experts').

As for the interobserver agreement observed in the 17 'novices' and the 19 'experts' the overall Kappa score suggests 'good' and 'excellent' agreement for the Gallstone Category; no statistically significant difference was noticed between the Kappa scores observed in the 2 groups.

According the the agreed criteria, intraobserver agreement was considered 'good' or 'excellent' in 35 of the 46 observers, 22 of whom showed 'perfect' agreement with previous readings on replicate ratings.

All the 46 observers rated the overall series into the four main diagnostic categories; some of them failed to rate a few cases of sludge and/or omitted to differentiate between single and multiple gallstones when appropriate. Hence, the self-selection of the observers could bias Kappa scores for interobservers' agreement on presence of sludge and number of gallstones.

The mean number of ratings per case of sludge was 29 (60% of total ratings); the Kappa score suggests 'good' interobserver agreement (K = 0.691).

Interobserver agreement beyond chance on the number of gallstones was calculated from the 25 'Gallstone Cases', i.e. rated as such by more than 90% of the raters. The mean number of ratings per case was 44 (96% of total ratings). Since gallstones could be rated into 3 categories (Single Gallstone; Multiple Gallstones; Number of Gallstones unassessable), the overall and category specific Kappa statistics were calculated.

The scores of the overall Kappa statistics suggest only a poor agreement on single gallstones (0.478).

Discussion

Although observers' variation has important implications in clinical practice [11] and suggestions have been made to take this issue into account in clinical decision-making [12], the peculiar features of multicenter epidemiologic studies stress its importance. The development of fixed criteria on both techniques and procedures to be employed for data collection and patients classification may prove insufficient, because of the adoption of unreliable criteria and/or their possible misuse by the observers.

Since a central panel to classify the 60 000 subjects enrolled in the multicenter Italian study on Epidemiology and Prevention of Cholelithiasis was not available, a study was performed to assess, and possibly improve, the quality of data.

Accuracy of the preliminary study was ensured through a careful selection of test images most likely to be observed in the field study. The overall levels of agreement between and within ultrasonographers observed in our study are as high as, or higher than those reported in clinical settings or in epidemiological studies using radiographs [13], electrocardiograms [14], endoscopy [15] or scintiscan [16]. Although they compare favourably with other diagnostic techniques, our results show that, despite the established criteria, the ultrasonographers' interpretation of the same image is neither the same nor constant over time.

Category specific Kappa scores suggest that observers are likely to agree on positive and negative cases, while agreement is poor on 'Doubtful' or 'Inconclusive' images. In fact, Doubtful and Inconclusive categories have been apparently used to overcome uncertainties in rating examinations into 'Gallstone' or 'No Gallstone' categories.

Kappa scores for the 'Gallstone' category are slightly higher than those observed for the 'No Gallstone' category. This does not agree with the available evidence suggesting that agreement is usually higher on negative diagnoses [17], and could be explained by the frequency of gallstone images in the videotape.

Although few studies addressed this point with conflicting results [18, 19], experienced observers are generally believed to be in agreement more often than less experienced observers. In our study, no difference was found between the overall and category specific Kappa scores between unexperienced and experienced ultrasonographers.

This does not mean that the observers were equally reliable in diagnosing gallstones, although both motivation and the established diagnostic criteria led novices to be as accurate as experts. Our results suggest that, in epidemiological studies, the observer's experience should not be overestimated as compared to other determinants of variation, such as feasibility and reliability of agreed criteria and type of rating required.

Disagreement in interpretation of clinical findings is a frequent issue in medicine, since inter- and intra-observer variation has always been found whenever it has been sought for [17, 20]. Our results suggest that, although established diagnostic criteria were adopted by trained ultrasonographers, their application may cause disagreement between and within observers. Hence, the crucial problems seem to be how to reduce variation and how to evaluate its impact on the study results.

Three main actions were taken to improve the quality of data: (1) a workshop was held to discuss the images most often disagreed upon in order to check the adequacy of their specific criteria: (2) ultrasonographers who performed poorly in the reliability study were offered further training; (3) a second reliability study was carried out, using a new series of cases focused on the major deficencies observed. Additionally, the code number of each ultrasonographer was recorded on the survey record, in order to analyze their individual performance.

References

1. Cooperberg PL, Burhenne HJ (1980): Real-time ultrasonography: diagnostic technique of choice in calculous gallbladder disease. *N Engl J Med* 302: 1277—1279.
2. Crade M, Taylor KJ, Rosenfield AT et al. (1978): Surgical and pathological correlation of cholecystosonography and cholecystography. *A J R* 131: 227—229.
3. Rabinowitz JG, Yeh HC, Cohen BA (1983): Gallstone update: Radiology. *Sem Liver Dis* 3: 120—131.
4. Rome Group for the Epidemiology and Prevention of Cholelithiasis (GREPCO) (1984): Prevalence of Gallstone Disease in an Italian Adult Female Population. *Am J Epidemiol* 118: 796—805.
5. Barbara L (1984): Epidemiology of gallstone disease: the 'Sirmione Study', pp. 23—25 in: Capocaccia L, Ricci G, Angelico F et al. (eds), *Epidemiology and Prevention of Gallstone Disease* Lancaster, MTP Press.
6. Barbara L, Festi D, Morselli Labate AM et al. (1984): Ultrasonography in the evaluation of the prevalence of gallstone disease: Progetto Sirmione, pp. 73—75 in: Labò G, Bolondi L, Rizzatto G (eds), *Clinical Advances in Ultrasonology* Masson.
7. McIntosh DMF, Penney HF (1980): Gray-scale ultrasonography as a screening procedure in the detection of gallbladder disease. Radiology 136: 725—727.

8. Fleiss JL (1981): *Statistical Methods for Rates and Proportions*, 2nd ed. New York, Wiley.

9. Fleiss JL (1971): Measuring nominal scale agreement among many raters. *Psychol Bull* 76: 378—382.

10. Landis JR, Koch CG (1977): The measurement of observer agreement for categorical data. *Biometrics* 33: 159—174.

11. Department of Clinical Epidemiology and Biostatistics, McMaster University: Clinical Disagreement (1980): I. How often it occurs and why. *Can Med Ass J* 123: 499—504.

12. Roberts CJ (1983): Evaluation of diagnostic services, pp. 176—188 in: Holland WW (ed), *Evaluation of Health Care* London: Oxford Univ. Press.

13. Geffen N, Darnborough A, De Dombal FT et al. (1968): Radiological signs of Ulcerative Colitis: Assessment of their reliability by means of observer variation studies. *Gut* 9: 150—156.

14. Acheson RM (1960): Observer error and variation in the interpretation of electrocardio-grams in an epidemiological study of coronary heart disease. *Brit J Prev Soc Med* 14: 99—122.

15. Conn HO, Smith HW, Brodoff M (1965): Observer variation in the endoscopic diagnosis of esophageal varices. *N Engl J Med* 272: 830—834.

16. Gjorup T, Brahm M, Fogh J et al. (1986): Interobserver variation in the detection of metastases on liver scans. *Gastroenterology* 90: 166—172.

17. Koran LM (1975): The reliability of clinical methods, data and judgements. *N Engl J Med* 293: 642—646; 695—701.

18. Allen-Mersh TG, Motson RW, Hately W (1985): Does it matter who does ultrasound examination of the gallbladder? *Brit Med J* 291: 389—390.

19. Nishiyama H, Lewis JT, Ashare AB et al. (1975): Interpretation of radionuclide liver images: do training and experience make a difference? *J Nucl Med* 16: 11—16.

20. Feinstein AR (1985): A bibliography of publications on observer variability. *J Chron Dis* 38: 619—632.

6. Prevalence of gallstone disease in 18 Italian population samples: first results from the MICOL study

THE MICOL GROUP*

Introduction

Although gallstone disease is recognized as a common disease, up to quite recently little evidence was available about its real prevalence and incidence in the general population. After early estimates of gallstone disease prevalence from autopsy studies, and clinically diagnosed cases of the disease [1—5], it was only with the advent of ultrasonography that epidemiological studies could be conducted on a large number of subjects with some degree of reliability. These include, among others, a few previous Italian studies [6—7].

The MICOL study (Multicenter Italian study on Epidemiology of Cholelithiasis) was designed to obtain a very large sample from the general population which would permit an overview of the distribution of gallstone disease in Italy for both sexes. Thus, 18 population samples of male and female subjects in ten Italian regions, were enrolled in the study, with a total population of about 54 000 individuals. The main results of this study, based on the cross-sectional part of the overall study, are reported in this paper.

Study design and methods

Eighteen centers agreed to participate in the study. Each center was to select a cohort of approximately 2000—2500 males and 1000—1500 females, aged 30—69 years. Such numbers were indentified on the basis of statistical power considerations. Once allowing for a proportion of non-participation of about 1/3, each sample would independently give, for each sex, prevalence estimates with a relative standard error of about 10% of the expected mean value. Furthermore, while testing the associations between factors and prevalence, these sample sizes would give a power of 0.8 to detect as significant, at the conventional probability level of 0.05, an odds ratio of 1.5

* For the composition of the MICOL group see p. xi (list of contributors).

L. Capocaccia et al. (eds), Recent advances in the epidemiology and prevention of gallstone disease, 37—44.
© 1991 *Kluwer Academic Publishers. Printed in the Netherlands.*

associated to a difference of one standard deviation in the independent variables.

A higher proportion of males was chosen in order to obtain a similar absolute number of cases in the two sexes due to the expected lower prevalence of gallstone disease (GD) in males than in females. The age range was chosen on the basis of previous experience suggesting that the overwhelming majority of cases falls within these limits.

Eighteen cohorts were selected by the participating centres by random sampling from the population registries of conveniently chosen municipalities. The distribution of all cohorts within Italy is shown in Fig. 1. Selected subjects were invited by mail to participate in a general program of preventive medicine, without any specific mention of gallstone disease. To

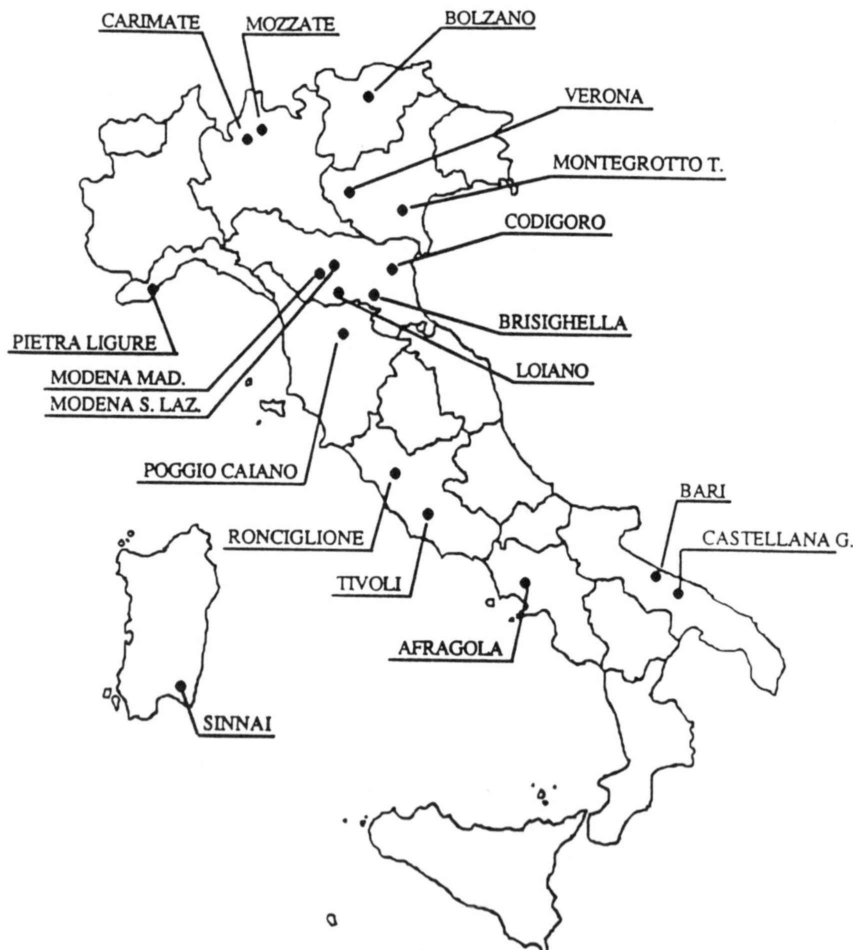

Fig. 1. Sites of the 18 MICOL cohorts.

maximize participation, conferences to inform the local population about the study were organized when possible, and general practitioners were contacted in order to obtain their support and collaboration. Non-respondents to the mailing invitation were contacted a second time either by mail or telephone.

Screening started in December, 1984 and terminated in April, 1987. Each subject filled in a precoded questionnaire, had a physical examination including anthropometric and blood pressure measurements, an ultrasonographic screening of the upper abdomen and a blood sampling for biochemical analyses.

The questionnaire was administered by a member of the medical staff. Questions regarded family and medical history, dietary habits, past and present use of drugs, with emphasis on cholesterol-lowering agents. Females were asked about menstrual cycle, number of pregnancies and use of oestroprogestinic drugs. Physical examination was also performed during the visit.

Quality control studies were carried out in order to test the reliability of ultrasonographic and chemical laboratory findings.

Each center was provided with the same ultrasonographic equipment, i.e. a real-time machine (Kontron, Mod Sigma 20) equipped with a 3.5 MHz linear transducer. Standardized criteria were established for both the examination and diagnosis. The inter- and intra-observer variation in the ultrasonographic detection of gallstones was assessed by means of a reliability study [8]. A standard oral cholecystography was also performed, when possible, for patients with an ultrasonographic diagnosis of gallstones. Findings relative to these examinations will not be reported here, as they are beyond the scope of this study.

To estimate the prevalence of gallstone disease, the final gallbladder status was recorded as follows: (1) Normal at ultrasonography; (2) Presence of gallstones at ultrasonography (GS); (3) Presence of biliary sludge at echography; (4) Previous cholecystectomy (CC). Gallstone disease (GD) was defined as conditions 2 or 4. The already mentioned paper [8] reports for ultrasonography a very good inter-observer agreement on definite presence or absence of GS diagnoses and less so for doubtful diagnoses.

A blood sample was obtained in the fasting condition for the measurement of glucose, total and high-density lipoprotein cholesterol, triglycerides, SGPT, gamma-glutamyltranspeptidase. A quality control on all biochemical analyses was performed under the supervision of the Biochemical Laboratory of the National Institute of Health, and for serum cholesterol, triglycerides, and glucose measurements shows non negligible between-laboratory effects. Regression analyses of obtained versus expected measures showed regression slopes generally bound between 0.9 and 1.1. Among the 16 laboratories of the centers belonging to the pooled sample, only three centers (b = 0.868, b = 0.888, and b = 1.151) for triglycerides and two centers (b = 1.196, and b = 0.685) for glucose, showed regression slopes outside these limits. The variability of the intercept, which is a measure of the mean laboratory error was more relevant.

This preliminary communication is concerned with the description of the prevalence of gallstone disease in the large population studied.

All subjects observed by the different centers were pooled together for most analyses, using the necessary caution to avoid geographical biases from this pooling procedure. Specifically, two types of analyses were implemented in order to detect possible sources of confounding. First of all, an analysis was carried out by means of a log-linear model expressing the probabilty of being a case as the product of two separated terms: the first depending on age, and the second on the specific cohort, and the significance of the cohort term was tested. Then, a regression on the mean age adjusted values of gallstone prevalence plotted against the values of each associated factor for all Units, was analyzed.

Results

A total of 33 699 out of the 54 040 enrolled subjects were actually examined, with an overall participation ratio of 62.0%. A small number of subjects — 105 males and 100 females — were not considered in the analysis due to the incompleteness of their ultrasonographic record. Participation was uniform over all age classes, slightly lower for males (60.7%) than for females (63.5%).

The number of invited subjects, the percentage of those with a clearcut final gallbladder status and the age adjusted prevalence of gallstones, cholecystectomy, or gallstone disease are shown in Table 1 for each center and for each sex. In the last row of the table the coefficients of variation of the prevalence, obtained by dividing the standard deviation of the reported values by their mean, are reported in order to give a measure of the degree of prevalence variability between cohorts. The reported figures show that geographical variability of the prevalence is high, and even more so for gallstones and cholecystectomy than for the combination of the two.

The data from all centers were then pooled together, controlling for possible confounding. Two Units (Florence and Naples) were excluded from the pool, due to the small number of invited subjects and very low participation. The remaining sixteen Units were tested for possible geographical association between their prevalence levels (gallstones + cholecystectomy) and participation ratios. The correlation coefficient between these two variables was not significantly different from zero both for males ($r = -0.08$) and for females ($r = -0.45$). We will refer to the sample obtained by pooling the data in the remaining 16 centers as to the 'pooled sample'.

The prevalence of gallstones, cholecystectomy, and both conditions, by age and sex in the pooled sample (consisting of 17 374 men and 14 817 women) is reported in Fig. 2. Standard errors of rates are not reported

Table 1. Number of individuals sampled and enrolled, percentage of respondents and prevalence of individuals with gallstones (GS), cholecystectomized (CC), and with either of the two conditions (GD), by sex and Operating Unit. Last row: coefficients of variation of the prevalence between Units.

| | Males | | | | | | Females | | | | | |
| | Enrolled | | | Prevalence | | | Enrolled | | | Prevalence | | |
Population	Sample	N	%	GS	CC	GD	Sample	N	%	GS	CC	GD
Bari	2743	1491	54	7.1	4.0	11.1	2057	1011	49	9.9	7.4	17.3
Lojano (BO)	1390	955	69	4.9	1.6	6.4	1246	874	70	9.0	6.3	15.3
Brisighella (BO)	1037	789	76	6.7	1.8	8.5	1040	823	79	9.5	6.0	15.5
Bolzano	1424	680	48	4.4	5.1	9.5	1200	598	50	8.2	12.5	20.7
Sinnai (CA)	2002	1093	55	7.7	0.9	8.6	1500	1054	70	18.9	5.3	25.2
Castellana (BA)	1885	1410	75	3.5	3.0	6.5	1431	1024	72	7.1	5.6	12.7
Mozzate (CO)	1080	884	82	4.8	3.2	8.0	1627	1029	63	9.3	10.5	19.8
Codigoro (FE)	1733	1205	70	7.9	4.2	12.1	1853	1282	69	8.1	9.9	18.0
Poggio Caiano (FI)	660	316	48	4.7	2.5	7.2	710	310	44	7.4	6.5	13.9
Carimate (CO)	903	622	69	6.7	3.2	9.9	821	659	80	8.8	8.2	17.0
Modena-S. Lazzaro	1951	1365	70	9.5	3.5	13.0	1455	1002	69	11.6	8.6	19.2
Modena-Madonnina	1997	1212	61	6.7	3.5	10.2	1510	932	62	10.5	10.6	21.1
Afragola (NA)	720	281	39	8.2	4.3	12.5	730	396	54	16.6	12.1	28.7
Montegrotto (PA)	2207	1337	61	4.4	1.8	6.2	1509	1096	73	9.7	7.0	16.7
P. Ligure etc. (SV)	2000	1069	53	9.0	2.7	11.7	1500	867	58	12.4	9.0	21.4
Tivoli (RM)	2313	1446	63	5.7	4.5	10.2	1856	1166	63	10.4	12.0	22.4
Ronciglione (RM)	2202	1118	51	4.9	1.7	6.6	1291	930	72	9.0	7.1	16.1
Verona	1335	698	52	6.7	5.2	11.9	1122	470	42	10.8	11.3	22.1
Total	29582	17971	60.7	6.3	3.1	9.4	24458	15523	63.5	10.6	8.6	19.2
Coeff. of Variation				0.27	0.41	0.24				0.29	0.28	0.21

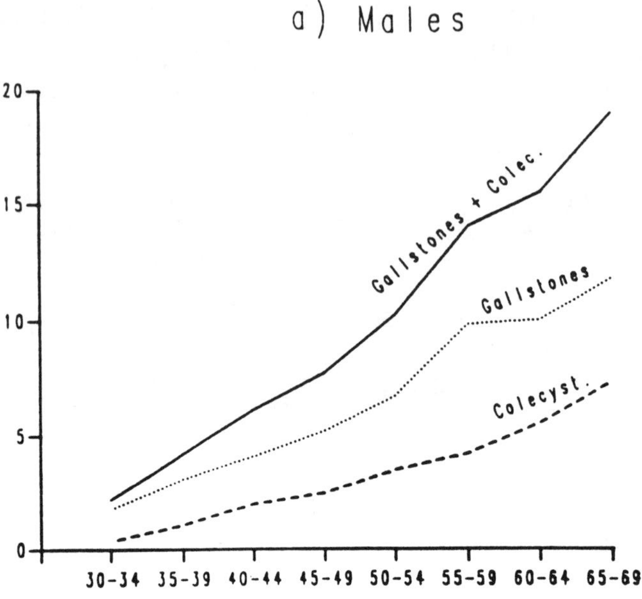

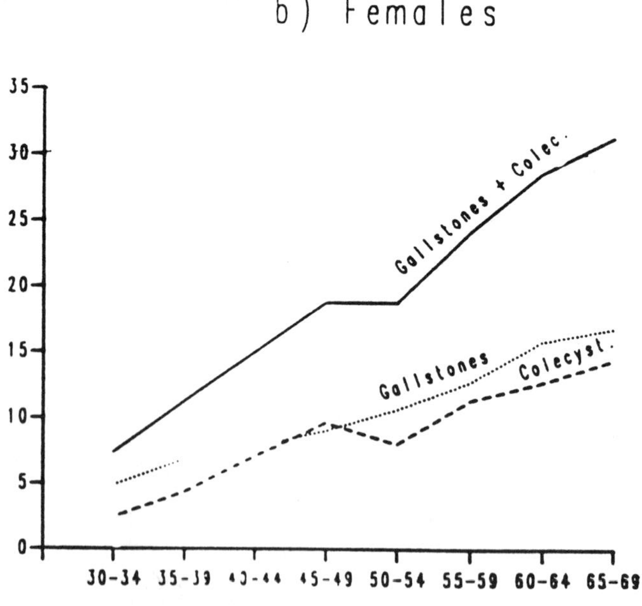

Fig. 2. Prevalence trends of gallstones and cholecystectomy with age (a) Males (b) Females.

because in no case they were very small when compared with the observed differences. For males, the mean prevalence of subjects with gallstones was 6.4%, and the overall proportion of cholecystectomized subjects was 3.1%. For females the corresponding figures were 10.4 and 8.6% respectively. It can be observed that (i) prevalence is higher for females than for males in all age groups; (ii) the female/male ratio is particularly high for cholecystectomy; (iii) for both sexes, the gallstones to cholecystectomy ratio is very high for young people, decreases with age, and approaches a value close to one for the oldest age groups (particularly for women).

Discussion

This study was not specifically designed as a survey aimed at obtaining prevalence estimates in a representative sample of the Italian population. The 18 municipalities from which the observed samples were taken — although spread over 10 out of the total 20 Italian regions — were selected for reasons of convenience, as they were near and accessible to the centers. However, within each municipality, subjects were invited to join the program by random sampling from the list of residents of the considered age group. As a consequence, study results most likely provide a comprehensive picture of gallstone disease prevalence levels and variability within the country.

The overall prevalence observed in the sample should not be much different from the value which would have been obtained in a true point estimate of disease occurrence in the whole population.

The overall participation ratio in the present study was lower than that obtained in previous epidemiological studies [6, 7] on gallstone disease performed in Italy. However, here the spreading of centers all over Italy did not allow to concentrate efforts on a single site and therefore was to some extent predictable. Of course, the possibility that participation bias might have influenced the results cannot be excluded in principle. However, a serious bias is unlikely to have occurred for several reasons.

First of all, in describing the programme to the invited subjects as a general program of preventive medicine, no mention was made of its specific goal.

Moreover, most of the prevalent subjects were unaware of having gallstones. After excluding the two cohorts with the lowest sample size, i.e. among the 16 cohorts contributing to the pooled sample, the correlation between participation and prevalence was negative for females and near zero for males. An interesting feature of the age trend of total prevalence is its marked linearity which suggests that age could be a variable correlated to the prevalence but not to the incidence of the disease. A recent incidence study on 89 000 U.S. women [9] based on mailed questionnaires reported a very weak relation of gallstone disease to age, when adjusted for relative weight. Of course, rates of increase in prevalence, measured at the same point in time, cannot be correctly interpreted as incidence rates, also for non fatal diseases, unless the absence of any relevant time trend can be assured. Prevalence increases with age by approximately 0.47% per year in males, and 0.67% per year in females. Increase rates in prevalence with age can be considered as an estimate of the difference between incidence rates and the unknown mean annual increase of disease occurrence. The higher value of the slope in females than in males can be probably attributed to the increase of the mean number of pregnancies with age.

It should be pointed out that these age trends, besides representing the mean trend, are actually representative of age trends in each of the sixteen cohorts of the pool. An analysis by means of a log-linear model yielded a satisfactory fit (X equal to 101 for males and 93 for females with 105 degrees of freedom) showing that there is no interaction between age and geographical area and indicating that all cohorts share the same sex-specific age trend.

References

1. Friedman GD, Kannel WB, Dawber TR (1966): The epidemiology of gallbladder disease: observations in the Framingham Study. *J Chron Dis* 19: 273—292.
2. Comess LJ, Bennett PH, Burch TA (1967): Clinical gallbladder disease in Pima Indians: its high prevalence in contrast to Framingham, Massachussets. *N Engl J Med* 277: 894—898.
3. Bennion LJ, Grundy SM (1978): Risk factors for the development of cholelithiasis in man. *N Engl J Med* 299: 1221—1227.
4. The Coronary Drug Project Research Group (1977): Gallbladder disease as a side effect of drugs influencing lipid metabolism. Experience in the Coronary Drug Project. *N Engl J Med* 296: 1185.
5. Layde PM, Vessey MP, Yeates D (1982): Risk factors for gallbladder disease: a cohort study of young women attending family planning clinics. *J Epidemiol Community Med* 36: 274—278.
6. Capocaccia L, Ricci G, Angelico F, Angelico M, Attili AF (eds) (1984): *Epidemiology and Prevention of Gallstone Disease.* MTP Press, Lancaster.
7. Barbara L, Sama C, Morselli Labate AM et al. (1987): A population study on the prevalence of gallstone disease: The Sirmione Study. *Hepathology* 7: 913—917.
8. Festi D, Lalloni L, Taroni F et al. (1989): Inter and Intra-observer variation in ultrasonographic detection of gallstones: The Multicenter Italian Study on Epidemiology of Cholelithiasis (MICOL). *Eur J Epidemiol* 5: 51—57.
9. Maclure KM, Hayes KC, Colditz GA et al. (1989): Weight, diet and the risk of symptomatic gallstones in middle-aged women. *N Engl J Med* 321: 563—569.

PART TWO

The natural history of gallstone disease

7. The natural history of gallstones: the GREPCO experience

A. F. ATTILI, R. CAPRI, A. M. REPICE, S. MASELLI,
and THE GREPCO GROUP*

Therapeutic decisions largely depend on our knowledge of the natural history of a disease. Most of the available data derive from clinical series of cases [1—7]. Only in one study [8] were 123 subjects identified as having gallstones by cholecystographic screening of a healthy population and followed prospectively for up to 20 years. These, however, were mainly white American faculty members of the University of Michigan and extrapolation of the results to the general population would be difficult.

A cohort of subjects with gallstones was identified by the Rome group for Epidemiology and Prevention of Cholelithiasis (GREPCO) between 1981 and 1984. A prospective follow-up was initiated, aimed at evaluating the clinical outcome of these subjects. The preliminary results of the prospective follow-up of initially asymptomatic subjects are reported here.

Methods

During the cross-sectional studies [9—11] performed by GREPCO, 161 civil servants (95 males and 66 females) were identified as having gallstones in their gallbladder. Most of these subjects were previously unaware of being a case, but they were informed about their presence when the diagnosis was made. Patients ranged in age between 27 and 69 yr. The recruitment period was between February 1981 and April 1982 for females and between December 1981 and July 1984 for males. The diagnosis was made on the basis of a positive ultrasonographic finding. A confirmative standard oral cholecystography was obtained in 100 subjects. Subjects were referred to their family doctor and no therapy was recommended by members of the study group. According to the criteria previously defined [12], 36 subjects were symptomatic (i.e. complained of at least one episode of biliary colic in the last 5 years) and 125 were asymptomatic. Prevalence of male sex was higher among asymptomatic (65.3%) than symptomatic (25%) subjects. We

* For the composition of the GREPCO group see p. x (list of contributors).

L. Capocaccia et al. (eds), Recent advances in the epidemiology and prevention of gallstone disease, 47—50.
© 1991 *Kluwer Academic Publishers. Printed in the Netherlands.*

will refer in this paper only to the data concerning the natural history of initially asymptomatic cases. We are prospectively following these subjects to determine the incidence of biliary colic, complications (acute cholecystitis, biliary obstruction or pancreatitis) and cholecystectomy. Data have been collected at least every two years with periodic follow-up evaluations at the appraisal unit. Precoded questionnaires were administered by members of the study group. Hospital records were examined in the occurrence of complications or cholecystectomy. Life table analysis was used in order to determine the cumulative probability of developing biliary colic, complications or being submitted to cholecystectomy. Subjects were considered to be at risk until they reached a definite end point (biliary colic, complication, death or cholecystectomy or the date of September 1989). Univariate and multivariate analysis models were used in order to determine whether some variables were capable of modifying the natural history of asymptomatic gallstones. The variables tested were: age, sex, awareness of having gallstones before diagnosis, number and diameter of gallstones, radioopaqueness, gallbladder opacification). The BMDP statistical package (Los Angeles, California, U.S.A.) was used.

Results

Nine (7.2%) of the 125 asymptomatic subjects included in the study were lost from the follow-up after the initial assessment. During the 5—8 yr follow-up period 8 subjects died, none for gallstone related causes or for gallbladder cancer. At the last follow-up visit (September 1989), 71 subjects were still asymptomatic, 24 had had at least one episode of biliary colic during the follow-up (in 12 cases biliary pain was severe enough to induce the patient to assume antispasmodics or to lie down), 1 subject developed an episode of acute cholecystitis after a one month period of biliary colic, 22 subjects had been submitted to cholecystectomy (12 prophylactic, 9 after at least one episode of biliary colic and 1 after the occurrence of an episode of acute cholecystitis). The life table analysis showing the occurrence of biliary colic or cholecystectomy is shown in Figs. 1 and 2, respectively. The mean survival time for biliary colic was 86.3 ($\pm$3.5 SE) months. The cumulative probability ($\pm$SE) of developing biliary colic was 12.3 $\pm$3.1 at 1 yr and at 2 yr, 17.3 $\pm$3.6 at 4 yr, 20.5 $\pm$4.1 at 6 yr. The mean survival time for cholecystectomy was 88.2 ($\pm$3.15 SE) months. The cumulative probability ($\pm$SE) of being submitted to cholecystectomy was 7.0 $\pm$2.4% at 1 yr, 10.6 $\pm$2.9 at 2 yr, 17.1 $\pm$3.5 at 4 yr and 19.8 $\pm$3.9 at 6 yr. None of the variables considered as possible modifiers of the natural history of asymptomatic gallstones were found to be associated with an increased risk of developing biliary colic or of being submitted to cholecystectomy.

Discussion

Despite their good reputation, there are many possible biases in prospective follow-up studies.

Firstly, misclassification of cases into the asymptomatic or the symptomatic groups might have occurred both at entry and during the follow-up. According to the definition of the GREPCO [9, 12], we considered as symptomatic those gallstone subjects who, in the last five years had complained of at least one episode of pain in the right hypocondrium or in the epigastrium lasting more than half an hour. Such a definition of biliary colic was accepted because gallstone females, in the first GREPCO study [9, 12] experienced this type of pain more frequently than subjects without gallstones. In gallstone men, however, presence of biliary pain, as previously defined, was not more frequent than in gallstone-free subjects [10]. According to Jorgensen [13], there is no symptom which clearly differentiates between subjects with gallstones and those without. We believe that our definition of biliary colic might, in the symptomatic group, include more false positive than false negative cases in the asymptomatic group. This could give rise to an abnormally high incidence of biliary colic during the follow-up.

The second possible bias could be due to the fact that most of the subjects included in the study were previously unaware of having gallstones. Once informed, they might have paid more attention to their symptoms, consulted their physician more frequently, changed their dietary habits, etc. The higher incidence of both biliary colic and cholecystectomy during the first two years of follow-up bears out the occurrence of such a bias in our study. This bias could have been avoided if subjects, identified as having gallstones, had not been informed about their presence. For ethical reasons, the steering committee of the GREPCO decided to inform the participating subjects on the results of the screening procedures. On the other hand, we wonder how it would have been possible to submit uninformed subjects to follow-up procedures such as cholecystography or gallbladder ultrasonography. A declining incidence of biliary colic was observed in at least two other studies [7, 14]. This observation, apart from the previously mentioned recall bias, might be explained by a selection of cases which are not prone to developing biliary pain during the follow-up.

The cumulative probability of developing biliary colic after 6 years of follow-up was much higher in the present study than in the Gracie and Ransohoff study (20.5 versus 10% respectively) [7]. The results, however, showed greater similarity (8.2 versus 10% respectively) when the incidence of biliary colic during the first year was subtracted from the overall incidence rate in both studies.

More than half of the subjects submitted to cholecystectomy during the follow-up were operated on in the absence of specific symptoms. This observation indicates that Italian physicians have an aggressive approach to the treatment of gallstones which is in contrast to the recommendations of an international Working Team published recently [15].

References

1. Comfort MW, Gray HK, Wilson JM (1948): The silent gallstone: a ten to twenty year follow-up study of 112 cases. *Ann Surgery* 128: 931—7.
2. Lund J (1960): Surgical indications in cholelithiasis: prophylactic cholecystectomy elucidated on the basis of long-term follow-up on 526 non-operated cases. *Ann Surgery* 151: 153—62.
3. Newman HF, Northup JD (1968): Complications of cholelithiasis. *Am J Gastroenterology* 50: 476—96.
4. McSherry CK, Ferstenberg H, Calhoun WF, Lahman E, Virshup M (1987): The natural history of diagnosed gallstone disease in symptomatic and asymptomatic patients. *Ann Surgery* 202: 59–63.
5. Ralston DE, Smith LA (1965): The natural history of cholelithiasis: a 15 to 30 year follow-up of 116 patients. *Minn Med* 48: 327—32.
6. Wenchert A, Robertson B (1986): The natural course of gallstone disease: an eleven year review of 781 non-operated cases. *Gastroenterology* 50: 376—81.
7. Thistle JL, Cleary MS, Lachin JM et al. (1984): The natural history of cholelithiasis: the National Cooperative Gallstone Study, *Ann Intern Med* 101: 171—75.
8. Gracie WA, Ransohoff DF (1982): The natural history of silent gallstones. The 'innocent' gallstone is not a myth. *N Engl J Med* 307: 798—800.
9. The Rome Group for the Epidemiology and Prevention of Cholelithiasis (GREPCO) (1984): Prevalence of gallstone disease in an Italian adult female population. *Am J Epidemiology* 119: 796—805.
10. The Rome Group for the Epidemiology and Prevention of Cholelithiasis (GREPCO) (1988): The epidemiology of gallstone disease in Rome, Italy. Part I. Prevalence data in men. *Hepatology* 8: 904—6.
11. Urbinati GC, the GREPCO (1984): Prevention of coronary heart disease and risk of cholelithiasis, pp. 193—8 in: Capocaccia L, Ricci G, Angelico F, Angelico M, Attili AF, (eds). *Epidemiology and Prevention of Gallstone Disease*, MTP Press, Lancaster.
12. Capocaccia, L, the GREPCO (1984): Clinical symptoms and gallstone disease: lessons from a population study, pp. 193—8 in: Capocaccia L, Ricci G, Angelico F, Angelico M, Attili AF (eds), *Epidemiology and Prevention of Gallstone Disease*, MTP Press, Lancaster.
13. Jorgensen T (1989): Abdominal symptoms and gallstone disease: an epidemiological investigation. *Hepatology* 9: 856—60.
14. Friedman GD, Raviola CA, Fireman B (1989): Prognosis of gallstones with mild or no symptoms: 25 years of follow-up in a health maintenance organization. *J. Clin. Epidemiol* 42: 127–36.
15. Shoenfield LJ, Carulli N, Dowling RH, Sama C, Wolpers C (1989): Asymptomatic gallstones: definition and treatment. *Gastroenterol Int* 2: 25—9.

8. Natural history of gallstone disease: the Sirmione study

C. SAMA, L. BARBARA, D. FESTI, R. FRABBONI,
A. M. MORSELLI LABATE, M. C. NACCHIERO, S. PARRO,
G. POLLINI, E. RODA, M. ROSSI, A. G. RUSTICALI, F. TARONI,
G. TASSINARI, C. BANTERLE, S. COLASANTI, G. FORMENTINI,
O. MORENI, F. NARDIN, M. C. PILIA and A. PUCI

In the past many textbooks have indicated that the onset of symptoms and biliary complications are the rule for patients with gallstones, and therefore cholecystectomy has been widely performed all over the world also in subjects with asymptomatic disease.

Over the past decade, however, some alternatives to cholecystectomy for the treatment of gallstone disease have become available (as dissolution with oral bile acids, lithotripsy and contact dissolution with solvents), and the wide-spreading use of ultrasonography has lead to the discovery of a large number of asymptomatic stones. Recent studies on epidemiology of gallstone disease have confirmed that the large majority of gallstones are silent [1, 2].

Some years ago a study from the University of Michigan [3], demonstrated that the natural history of asymptomatic gallstones, as a matter of fact, is a fairly benign disease, and stimulated a change in the therapeutic approach to the disease and a number of studies on the natural history of gallstone disease.

Evaluation of the natural history of gallstone disease requires, however, careful definition of the population at risk, a large cohort of subjects and prolonged periods of surveillance. Out of the large literature which exists on the argument, only few studies fulfill these criteria.

If we consider the patients with symptomatic stones, i.e. patients with biliary symptoms or a history of biliary symptoms (Table 1), we can see that most of them have recurrence of symptoms and that many develop biliary complications. The risk of development of complications is higher if the patient has frequent and severe symptoms [4]. If we consider subjects with truly asymptomatic disease (i.e. those patients who never experienced biliary symptoms) the natural history of gallstone disease seems to be more benign (Table 2). In fact the available studies show that in a time period ranging from 5 to 24 years the yearly incidence of biliary pain varies from 0.5 to 4%.

Because of the controversies that still exist in this field, one of the purposes of the Sirmione study [1] was the evaluation of the natural history of gallstone cases detected during the study itself.

L. Capocaccia et al. (eds), Recent advances in the epidemiology and prevention of gallstone disease, 51–55.
© 1991 *Kluwer Academic Publishers. Printed in the Netherlands.*

52   *C. Sama et al.*

Table 1. Symptomatic gallstone disease: natural history.

Author	No. of subjects	Years of follow-up	Incidence rate (%)	
			Biliary pain and complications	Complications
Lund [4]	201	5—20	58	27
Ralston [5]	71	15—30	68	nr
Wenckert [6]	781	1—11	33	18
Gomand [7]	40	8—17	72	28

Table 2. Asymptomatic gallstone disease: natural history.

Author	No. of subjects	Years of follow-up	Incidence rate (%)	
			Biliary pain and complications	Complications
Comfort [8]	112	10—20	19	4.4
Ralston [5]	14	15—30	29	nr
Newman [9]	191	2—22	10	nr
Gracie [3]	123	11—24	16	1
McSherry [10]	135	3.8[a]	10.4	2

[a] Median.

In 1982 during the first cross-sectional study, 132 cases have been identified. The study protocol included a questionnaire inquiring as to the presence of gallstones and/or previously cholecystectomy, as well as to the presence of both specific and non-specific biliary symptoms. In our study subjects were defined as having specific biliary symptoms if they suffered, during the last 5 years, from abdominal pain, in the right upper abdomen or epigastrium, which had lasted for more than half an hour and was not relieved by bowel movements. The occurrence of non-specific symptoms (nausea, bloating, upper abdominal discomfort, headache and irregular bowel habits) was also inquired about.

Twenty-nine (21.9%) out of the 132 subjects proved to have gallstones in their gallbladder at the time of the study, had suffered from biliary pain in the 5 yr before the interview, versus 2.4% of subjects without gallstones ($X^2 = 128$; $P < 0.001$). No difference was observed either in number or frequency of non-specific symptoms between subjects with and without gallstones (Fig. 1).

Silent stones, defined as gallstones that had not caused biliary pain or complications, accounted for 78% of the 132 cases; of the 24 cases who were aware of having stones prior to the study, 9 had silent stones (Fig. 2).

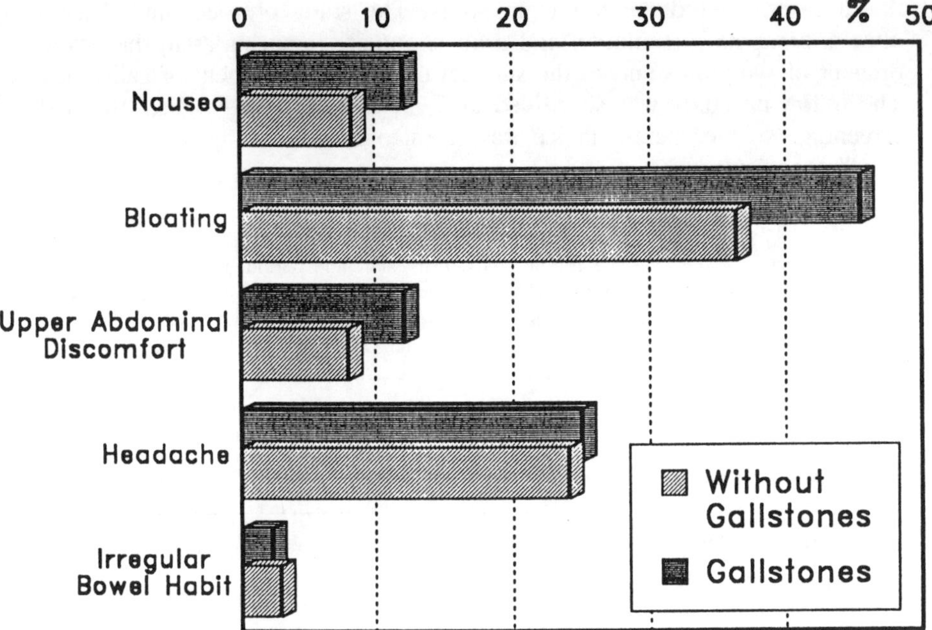

Fig. 1. Occurrence of non specific symptoms (%) in subjects with and without gallstones. Frequency of each symptom was not significantly different in gallstone vs. non gallstone subjects.

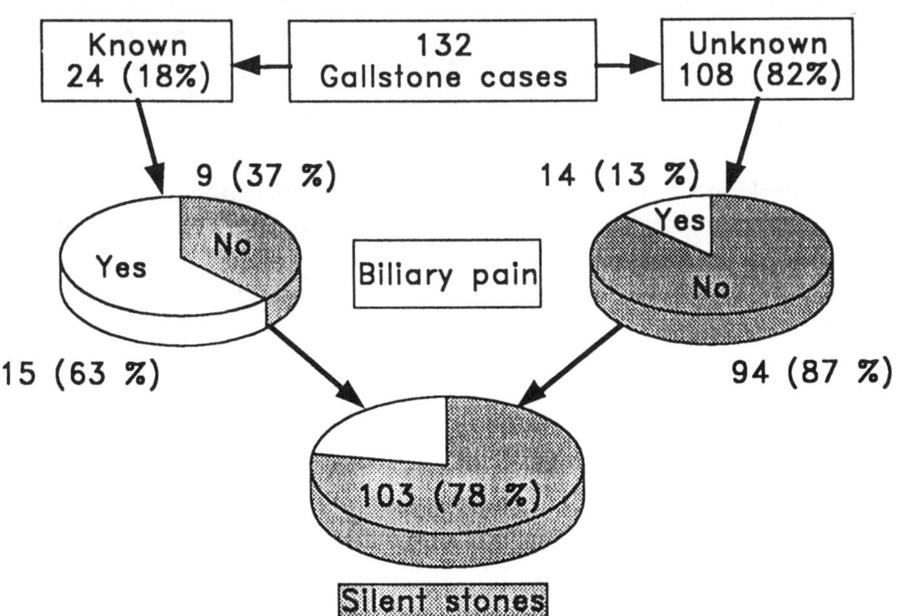

Fig. 2. Gallstone cases observed in the Sirmione study in relation to the frequency of biliary symptoms and awareness of the disease prior to the study.

All cases entered the follow-up study. The study protocol included an ultrasonographic examination and a questionnaire inquiring as to the development of symptoms and to the surgical or medical treatment of gallstones. The follow-up study was scheduled at 2, 3, 5, 8, and 10 yr after the first screening. No therapeutic advice was given to gallstone subjects at the time of gallstone detection.

Results at the fifth year are summarized in Table 3.

Table 3. Results of the five-year follow study. For each time period, the number of both observed and lost subjects, frequency of development of symptoms, and cholecystectomy rate are reported. Data are grouped according to the absence (Asymp) and the presence (Symp) of symptoms during the 5 years before the first observation in 1982.

Yr	Observed		Lost and drop-out		Symptoms cholecystectomy (% in the time-interval)			
	Asymp	Symp	Asymp	Symp	Asymp	Symp	Asymp	Symp
2	101	29	2	0	5.9	27.6	17.8	27.6
3	101	29	0	0	8.7	11.4	9.9	0
5	82	22	19	7	1.3	9.8	3.3	4.1
Cumulative percentage					15.9	48.8	31.0	31.7

X-ray visualization of gallbladder, size, number and composition of stones were not predictive factors for development of symptoms. Forty subjects with gallstones have been cholecystectomized during the follow-up period. Interestingly 20 subjects in the asymptomatic group underwent surgery being still asymptomatic. Two subjects out of the symptomatic group experienced biliary complications (mild pancreatitis and jaundice) and underwent surgery.

In conclusion a relatively high rate of development of symptoms in previously asymptomatic subjects has been observed in Sirmione during 5 years of follow-up (15.9%); however most symptoms have been observed during the first 2 yr and a much slower rate has been observed thereafter. Persistence or recurrence of symptoms have been observed in about 50% of previously symptomatic subjects.

References

1. Barbara L, Sama C, Morselli Labate AM, Taroni F, Rusticali AG, Festi D, Sapio C, Roda E, Banterle C, Puci A, Formentini F, Colasanti S, Nardin F (1987): A population study on the prevalence of gallstone disease: The Sirmione Study. *Hepatology* 7: 913—917.
2. GREPCO (1984): Prevalence of gallstone disease in an Italian adult female population. *Am J Epidemiol* 119: 796—805.
3. Gracie WA, Ransohoff DF (1982): The natural history of gallstones; the innocent gallstone is not a myth. *N Engl J Med* 307: 798—800.

4. Lund J (1960): Surgical indications in cholelithiasis. *Ann Surg* 151: 153—162.
5. Ralston DE, Smith LA (1965): The natural history of cholelithiasis: a 15 to 30-year follow-up of 116 patients. *Minn Med* 48: 327—332.
6. Wenckert A, Robertson B (1966): The natural course of gallstone disease: eleven-year review of 871 nonoperated cases. *Gastroenterology* 50: 376—381.
7. Gomand L, Vandenbroncke J, De Groote J (1966): Die natuurlijke evolutie van colelithiase. *Tijdschr Gastroenterol* 9: 594—601.
8. Comfort MW, Gray HK, Wilson JM (1948): The silent gallstone: a ten to twenty year follow-up study of 112 cases. *Ann Surg* 128: 913.
9. Newman HF, Northup JD, Rosenblum M, Abrams M (1968): Complications od cholelithiasis. *Am J Gastroenterol* 50: 476—496.
10. McSherry CK, Ferstenberg H, Colhoum WF, Lahman E, Virship M (1985): The natural history of diagnosed gallstone disease in symptomatic and asymptomatic patients. *Ann Surg* 202: 59—63.

9. The outcome of gallstone disease in symptomatic and asymptomatic patients

C. K. McSHERRY

Opportunities to study the natural history of gallstone disease are infrequent and also difficult to accomplish. Factors that contribute to the latter are the imprecise risk factors for the development of the disease, the often long latency period between the presence of stones and the onset of symptoms and the clinical difficulties associated with an accurate diagnosis of upper abdominal gastrointestinal disease. For many years, patients with gallstones, symptomatic or silent, were urged to undergo prompt cholecystectomy thus depriving epidemiologists the opportunity to study the course of the disease.

In the older literature, Moynihan [1] in 1908 and Mayo [2] in 1911 warned of the consequences of silent stones. Mayo wrote that the 'innocent' gallstone is a myth. In 1948, Comfort, Gray and Wilson [3] reported that 46% of patients with silent stones developed symptoms when followed from 10 to 20 yr. However, these authors included dyspepsia as a symptom of biliary calculi and, therefore, probably reported an artificially high incidence of symptoms directly attributable to gallstone disease. In 1960, Lund [4] reported on a group of 562 patients with cholelithiasis observed for from 5 to 20 yr. Of this group, 50% of the women and 30% of the men had symptoms of biliary calculous disease, usually within 5 yr of the diagnosis. The complications of gallstone disease, viz acute cholecystitis and jaundice, occurred in 25% of the patients. There did not appear to by any significant difference in prognosis between asymptomatic and symptomatic patients in this series. Wenkert and Robertson [5] followed 781 patients with cholelithiasis for 1 to 11 yr, and 33% developed symptoms, 18% jaundice of pancreatitis, and 5% acute cholecystitis.

In recent years, the need to reevaluate the fate of patients with silent stones was prompted by the report of Gracie and Ransohoff [6]. In 1982, these authors reported on 123 faculty members at the University of Michigan with asymptomatic gallstones. None of these individuals died because of gallstone disease, and the 15-year cumulative probability of the development of biliary symptoms or complications was only 18%. This report was viewed with some skepticism because the study group consisted almost entirely of white American males; only 13 of the 123 subjects were female.

L. Capocaccia et al. (eds), Recent advances in the epidemiology and prevention of gallstone disease, 57—63.
© 1991 *Kluwer Academic Publishers. Printed in the Netherlands.*

The present study was carried out in an effort to determine the natural history of gallstone disease in a population more representative of the American people.

Patient selection

The population reported herein are all members of the Health Insurance Plan of Greater New York (HIP). Established in 1947, HIP is the oldest prepaid group practice plan and the largest health maintenance organization in the Eastern United States. The medical and hospital care of its 900 000 subscribers is provided through nine affiliated medical group partnerships or professional corporations located throughout the Greater New York City and Northern New Jersey area. The plan has traditionally appealed to municipal employees and members of various unions representing a cross-section of middle income people of diverse ethinic origin. The availability of medical records containing both inpatient and outpatient data maintained in many instances for periods of several decades made this population ideal for this study. In addition, the absence of economic incentives for the HIP physicians to recommend or perform biliary tract surgery on the subscribers was another principal factor for choosing this group of patients. For logistical reasons, the records of the patients reported herein were chosen from three of the HIP centers in the borough of Queens. Although demographic data are unavailable for each of the HIP centers, we assume that the patients treated in these three centers are similar to those encountered throughout the HIP system. Each center provides medical and surgical care for patients of all ages.

The records of the adult patients at these three centers were reviewed for evidence of calculous biliary tract disease and its sequellae, which were confirmed and documented by such evidence as reports of radiographic or ultrasound examination and pathology or operative reports. At least 6 months elapsed from the date of diagnosis to operation, or in the non-operated patients, follow-up visits.

Symptomatology

The severity of the patients' symptoms were graded on a scale of 0 to +++. Patients with gastrointestinal symptoms or abdominal complaints that were ascribed to diseases other than biliary calculi were graded as zero. Patients that reported infrequent episodes of biliary colic, i.e. at intervals greater than monthly, had no evidence of acute cholecystitis or obstructive jaundice, and had their diagnostic studies performed as outpatients were considered +. Those patients with frequent episodes of biliary colic, usually at intervals of one month or less, of such severity as to require the parenteral use of analgesics and some loss of work-time were categorized as ++. Acute cholecystitis, evidenced by fever, leukocytosis and often hospitalization with or without obstructive jaundice, merited a +++. Similarly, obstructive jaundice in the absence of acute cholecystitis also resulted in +++ classification.

There were 691 patients that fulfilled the criteria for inclusion in this study: 450 (65.1%) females and 241 (34.9%) males. The racial distribution was 542 (78.4%) Caucasian; 112 (16.2%) Black; 35 (5.1%) Hispanic; and two (0.3%) Oriental. Their mean ± SD age was 65.5 ± 16.1 yr, with a range of 21 to 97 yr. The mean ± SD duration of observation from the date of diagnosis of calculous biliary tract disease to death or date of last contact was 78 ± 61.8 months, with range of 6.6 months to 33.3 yr (median 62.9 months).

Symptoms compatible with biliary tract disease were reported by 556 (80.5%) patients, and 135 (19.5%) were asymptomatic. Table 1 lists the type and frequency of the symptoms reported in the former group.

Table 1. The type and frequency of symptoms in 556 patients with gallstones.

Symptoms	Frequency (%)
Pain	540 (97.1)
Fatty food intolerance	206 (37.1)
Vomiting	81 (14.6)
Jaundice	43 (7.7)
Hemolytic anemia	7 (1.0)
Ileal disease	2 (0.3)

In the majority of symptomatic patients, the diagnosis of gallstone disease was confirmed by oral cholecystography. This roentgenographic study was performed in 519 (93.3%) of the 556 patients with symptoms. In 286 (51.4%) of the 556 symptomatic patients studied, functioning gallbladders that contained calculi were evident. In the other 233 (41.9%) patients, calculous disease was inferred on the basis of two consecutive studies that failed to visualize the gallbladder. Ultrasound examinations were performed in 94 (16.8%) patients, and gallstones were positively identified in 88 and suspected in an additional six. Radiopaque calculi were noted on plain roentgenograms of the abdomen in 60 (10.9%) patients. In 26 (4.6%) patients, intravenous cholangiograms were diagnostic of stone disease. In contrast, the majority or 87 (64.4%) of the 135 asymptomatic patients had radiopaque stones noted on roentgenograms of the abdomen performed as part of diagnostic studies for suspected nonbiliary intraabdominal diseases. Oral cholecystograms were performed in 80 asymptomatic patients to confirm the location of opaque calculi, or as part of comprehensive diagnostic evaluations. In 59 of these patients, the gallbladder functioned as evidenced by contrast within the lumen of this stricture. In 21, there was no opacification of the gallbladder. Ultrasound examination was performed in 23 (16%) patients and was positive in 21 and equivocal in two.

The mean and SD age of the asymptomatic patients was 73.6 ± 13.9 yr and the symptomatic group 63.6 ± 16.0 yr. This age difference is significant at $p < 0.0001$, using the 2-tail Student's t-test. In addition, there were proportionately more males in the asymptomatic group, 57 of 135 (42.4%), in comparison to the symptomatic group, 184 of 556 (33%). In addition to their advanced age, asymptomatic patients were also more ill than their symptomatic counterparts. The frequency of severe cardiovascular disease, New York Heart Association [7] Class 3 or 4, was 23.7% in the asymptomatic group and 7.9% in the symptomatic. Similarly the incidence of hypertension, blood pressure greater than 140/90, was 44.4% in the asymptomatic patients versus 27.8% in the symptomatic. The incidence of malignant disease, diabetes mellitus, hiatus hernia and duodenal ulcer was also higher in asymptomatic patients.

In the group of 556 patients with symptomatic biliary tract disease, physicians recommended operative therapy for 289 (52%). In 267 (48%) patients, surgery was not advised. The rationale behind these decisions was usually not evident from the medical records. The mean duration of follow-up to last contact in this group of patients was 82.9 ± 63.2 months (median 68.5 months). In symptomatic patients, the severity of symptoms at the time of diagnosis was categorized as + in 223 (40.1%) of the 556. Over the time span of this study, the intensity of symptoms was unchanged in 116 (52%), increased to ++ in 89 (39.9%), and +++ in 18 (8.1%). Thus, in slightly more than one-half of the patients (52%) with minimal (+) symptoms, the severity of their complaints remain unchanged. In the others (48%), symptoms increased. There were 145 (26.1%) patients whose symptoms were graded as ++ at the time of diagnosis, and in 69 (47.6%), the severity of these symptoms was unchanged immediately prior to operation or at the time of their last visit to the health center if they were not operated on. In 42 (29%), the severity of complaints decreased to +, and in one patient, completely subsided. In 33 (22.8%) patients, symptoms progressed to +++. Of the 188 (33.8%) patients with severe (+++) symptoms at the time of diagnosis, 29 (15.3%) continued at this level. In 42 (22.2%) the severity of symptoms decreased to ++, and in 116 (61.7%), +. One patient eventually became asymptomatic.

In this group of 556 symptomatic patients, biliary tract operations were eventually performed in 242 (43.5%). The mean duration from diagnosis to operation was 49.2 ± 53.6 months (median 31.3 months). The indications for operation were chronic cholecystitis and cholelithiasis in 189 (79%), nine of whom were jaundiced and acute cholecystitis in 47 (21%), 10 of whom were also jaundiced. Three patients had cholecystectomy incidental to other intraabdominal operations, and three had miscellaneous reasons for biliary tract surgery. Only one patient eventually developed carcinoma of the gallbladder. Cholecystectomy was performed in 234 (97%) patients, 49 of whom also had a choledochotomy. Stones were recovered from the common bile duct in 36 of these patients. Six patients underwent choledochoduodenostomy and two, cholecystostomy. The remaining 314 (56.3%) symptomatic patients were not operated on. The mean duration in months from the date of diagnosis to last known contact is 68.6 ± 56.6 months (median 53.9 months). In this group of patients, there were two (0.8%) postoperative deaths. There were 23 additional patients with symptomatic calculous disease that died of nonbiliary tract causes.

The patient that eventually proved to have carcinoma of the gallbladder is a 73-yr-old diabetic woman who experienced jaundice in 1976. Gallstones were evident on plain roentgenograms of the abdomen and untrasound studies. She refused to be operated on until 1980. The resected gallbladder contained stones and incidental carcinoma. She is alive and well at the present time.

Cholecystectomy was recommended to only seven (5.2%) of the 135 asymptomatic patients at the time of diagnosis, and none of these patients agreed to immediate operation. The mean and SD of the duration of follow-up in this group of patients was 58 ± 50.2 months (median 46.3 months). During this time interval, only 14 (10.4%) of the patients developed symptoms. The severity of symptoms in these 14 patients was + in five, ++ in five, and +++ in four. Three of these patients had acute cholecystitis, one of whom also had jaundice. One patient with chronic cholecystitis also had choledocholithiasis. Fifteen patients in this group inderwent biliary tract operations during the time span of this study. Five of these procedures consisted of a cholecystectomy performed incidental to another intraabdominal operation. Eight patients had a planned cholecystectomy, and one each, cholecystostomy and cholecystectomy plus common bile duct exploration. Six patients who developed symptoms of chronic cholecystitis and cholelithiasis were not operated on. Thus, the proportion of patients with asymptomatic stones that were operated on for biliary tract disease was 7.4%, or 10 of 135 patients. The time interval between diagnosis and operation in these 10 patients was 46.8 ± 55.4 months (median 24.9 months). There were no operative deaths and only one nonbiliary tract complication in these 10 patients. During this same time interval, 25 (18.5%) of the 135 asymptomatic patients died of nonbiliary tract disease.

The relationship of gallbladder function on oral cholecystography and the indications for cholecystectomy were examined in these patients. Of the 691 symptomatic and asymptomatic patients, 234 had oral cholecystography and eventually were operated on. In 151 patients there was sufficient contrast agent in the gallbladder to permit its visualization, and in the remaining 83 patients, the gallbladder did not visualize. In the former group, 19 (12.6%) were operated on for acute cholecystitis and 132 (87.4%), chronic cholecystitis. In the patients with nonvisualization of the gallbladder, 25 (30.1%) had acute cholecystitis and 58 (69.9%), chronic cholecystitis. These differences in the incidence of acute and chronic cholecystitis in relation to gallbladder function are statistically significant at p = 0.001.

In the symptomatic patients, the predictive value of gallbladder function on oral cholecystography with respect to outcome was also evaluated. Oral cholecystograms were obtained in 519 of 556 symptomatic patients, and the gallbladder visualized in 286 (55.1%) and failed to visualize in 233 (44.9%). In the patients whose gallbladder visualized, 149 (52.1%) were operated on and 137 (47.9%) were not operated on in the follow-up period. In contrast, in the group of patients with non-visualization of the gallbladder, 85 (36.5%) were operated on and 148 (63.5%) were not operated on for biliary tract disease. These differences with respect to gallbladder visualization and the proportion of patients operated on are significant at p = 0.0004. A similar analysis in asymptomatic patients was not possible because of the smaller number of patients in this category. Thus, it appears that patients with nonvisualization of the gallbladder are less likely to be operated on than their counterparts with a visualized gallbladder. However, if operated on, they are more likely to have acute cholecystitis than those patients with a visualized gallbladder on oral cholecystography.

Discussion

This report describes the long-term consequences of both asymptomatic and symptomatic gallstones. The optimal treatment of patients with asymptomatic stones has been controversial. Surgeons, in general, have advocated early removal of the gallbladder because of the higher mortality and morbidity rates of cholecystectomy in the older age group, and in those patients with acute cholecystitis and common duct obstruction. Internists, confronted with the patient with silent stones, usually do not recommend operation since, in many patients cholecystectomy will never prove necessary.

This study confirms the report of Gracie and Ransohoff [6] in a different and more heterogenious population. The onset of symptoms in our series of 135 patients was only 10.4%, and biliary tract operations were required in but 7.4%. Thus, patients with asymptomatic gallstones can be followed by their physicians with reasonable safety.

Information concerning patients with symptoms attributed to calculous biliary tract disease, but not operated on, is for the most part fragmentary and anecdotal. This report suggests that in patients with minimal symptoms observed for a mean time span of 64.5 ± 65.7 months, one-half will continue to have minimal symptoms and the other half an increase in the severity of their symptoms. In patients with symptoms graded as moderate, about one half continue at this level of intensity, one-quarter decrease, and one-quarter increase in severity. In patients with severe symptoms, the majority (approximately 85%) improved. Presumably, most of those individuals with severe persistant symptoms were operated upon in less than 6 months and are, therefore, not included in this study.

It is of consideragle interest that only 44% of symptomatic patients underwent operation. The reasons for this are many, but must include such factors as individual pain tolerance, fear of hospitalization and surgery, and failure of physicians to offer cholecystectomy as a reasonable therapeutic approach to gallstone disease.

In this series of 691 patients, there were only two biliary tract related deaths. The other 48 deaths that occurred in the time span of this study were from unrelated causes. In addition, only one patient developed carcinoma of the gallbladder, thus negating this factor as a meaningful argument in support of operative therapy.

The relatively infrequent need for cholecystectomy, even in symptomatic patients, suggests that many of these individuals with cholesterol stones can be considered as reasonable candidates for alternate therapies such as bile acid therapy and extra-corporeal shock wave lithotripsy.

References

1. Monihan BGA (1908): An address on inaugural symptoms. *Br Med J* 2: 1597—1601.
2. Mayo WJ (1911): Innocent gallstones a myth. *JAMA* 56: 1021—4.
3. Comfort MW, Gray HK, Wilson JM (1948): The silent gallstone: a ten to twenty year follow-up study of 112 cases. *Ann Surg* 128: 931—7.
4. Lund J (1960): Surgical indications in cholelithiasis: prophylactic cholecystectomy elucidated on the basis of long-term follow-up on 526 nonoperated cases. *Ann Surg* 151: 153—62.
5. Wenckert A, Robertson B (1966): The natural course of gallstone disease: eleven year review of 781 nonoperated cases *Gastroenterology* 50: 376—81.
6. Gracie WA, Ransohoff DF (1982): The natural history of silent gallstones. The innocent gallstone is not a myth. *N Engl J Med* 307: 798—800.
7. New York Heart Association Criteria Committee (1964): Diseases of the Heart and Blood Vessels. Nomenclature and Criteria for Diagnosis, 6th ed. Boston, Little, Brown & Co, 112.

10. Factors affecting the decision to undergo cholecystectomy for mildly symptomatic gallstones

G. D. FRIEDMAN

Elective cholecystectomy for the removal of gallstones is a frequently performed operation in Western societies [1, 2]. Recent analyses [3–6] suggest that either having or not having this operation electively makes little difference in average long-term survival for patients with gallstones. Thus, the decision to have a cholecystectomy depends on the level of enthusiasm of the physician and patient toward the procedure. The patient is strongly influenced, of course, by the severity of his or her symptoms that are attributed to the gallstones. However, this is clearly not the only factor affecting the decision because many patients with frequent or severe symptoms avoid cholecystectomy or delay it as long as possible and others with no symptoms readily accept the operation when it is recommended.

Little is known about characteristics of patients, other than their symptoms, that affect decisions about cholecystectomy. We recently completed a study of the prognosis of gallstones with mild or no symptoms [6]. Some of the study subjects had received multiphasic health checkups [7], at which extensive data about personal characteristics were collected by self-administered questionnaires. For this report, selected data were analyzed in the hope of identifying characteristics that would differentiate patients with mildly symptomatic gallstones who did, from those who did not, undergo cholecystectomy during the follow-up period of the study.

Methods

This study was conducted in the setting of the Kaiser Permanente Medical Care Program which provides prepaid medical care, both inpatient and outpatient, to about one quarter of the population of the San Francisco Bay Area. Subscribers are heterogenous, both ethnically and socioeconomically. In the study of the prognosis of gallstones [6], 298 patients with gallstones accompanied by mild or nonspecific symptoms, who could be followed up in records of the program, were identified in two computer-stored data sets. Follow-up duration ranged from less than one year to 37 years after diagnosis

L. Capocaccia et al. (eds), Recent advances in the epidemiology and prevention of gallstone disease, 65–70.
© 1991 *Kluwer Academic Publishers. Printed in the Netherlands.*

of gallstones. Of these patients, 41 developed severe complications during follow-up and were excluded from the present analysis. Of the remaining 257, 58 had a cholecystectomy during follow-up with various degrees of mild to moderate chronic symptoms occurring before surgery and 199 had no cholecystectomy during follow-up. Forty-eight (82.8%) of these 58 patients with cholecystectomy and 146 (73.4%) of these 199 without, had had a multiphasic health checkup at or before their 'index date,' which was the date at which the first indication that they might have gallstones appeared in our computer-stored records. (This date was usually later than the date of initial diagnosis of gallstones). Comparisons based on checkup questionnaire data had to be restricted to the latter 48 and 146 patients with and without cholecystectomy, respectively.

The mean length of follow-up from diagnosis until cholecystectomy was 6.4 yr for the 58 patients with this operation and 6.7 yr for the subset of 48 with checkup data. For the 199 and 146 corresponding patients without cholecystectomy, mean follow-up in our records was 13.2 and 14.4 yr, respectively. Thus, the non-operated patients were not lacking cholecystectomy because of having less follow-up time, on average, than the operated group.

Data items analyzed were selected to represent demographic characteristics, general health status, lifestyle, emotional status, and attitude concerning medical care. Statistical significance testing was accomplished by the chi-square test for categorical variables and the t-test for continuous variables.

Results

The patients who underwent cholecystectomy for mild symptoms were more apt to be women and tended to be younger at time of diagnosis than those who did not (Table 1). There were no significant differences in race, education or marital status.

At the checkup approximately equal percentages of the operated (33.3%) and non-operated (37.7%) patients reported some disability that limited their usual work or activity. The patients with cholecystectomy more often reported complete disability for work — 25.0% versus 15.8% — whereas the opposite was true for partial disability — 8.3% versus 21.9%. The overall comparison of responses to this question was of borderline statistical significance (p = 0.07). The distribution of reasons for having the checkup, selected from a five-choice question ('didn't feel well', 'regular annual checkup', 'wanted a checkup', 'doctor suggested it', 'someone else suggested it'), did not differ significantly between the two groups (p = 0.64).

Cigarette smoking was more prevalent among persons who underwent surgery. There was no significant difference in reported use of alcohol or reported eating or drinking to excess (Table 2).

There was no significant difference in the percentage of patients respond-

Table 1. Demographic characteristics of gallstone patients with mild symptoms who did and did not later undergo cholecystectomy. Age and sex comparisons were based on 58 of the former and 199 of the latter. All other comparisons are based on 48 of the former and 146 of the latter who had multiphasic health checkups.

	Cholecystectomy	None	p
Mean age at diagnosis (yr)	50.9	55.5	<0.01
Female sex (%)	84.5	71.4	0.04
Skin color			
white (%)	85.4	77.4	
black (%)	12.5	12.3	0.30
other (%)	2.1	10.3	
Education			
any college (%)	14.6	14.4	
no college (%)	85.4	85.6	0.78
Marital status			
currently married (%)	64.6	52.1	
never married (%)	22.9	31.5	0.32
divorced, widowed, separated (%)	12.5	16.4	

Table 2. Lifestyle habits reported at multiphasic health checkups by gallstone patients with mild symptoms who did and did not later undergo cholecystectomy.

	Cholecystectomy		None		
	Total No. responding	% yes	Total No. responding	% yes	p
Past year, smoke cigarettes	39	38.5	136	22.1	0.04
Past year, drink any alcohol	39	38.5	136	33.1	0.53
Usually eat and drink more than					
is good for you	40	20.0	136	12.5	0.23

ing who considered themselves to be 'the worrying type' — 33.3% of 30 operated and 35.1% of 97 non-operated (p = 0.86). This was also true for the self-report of 'often being unhappy and depressed' — 15.8% of 38 operated and 19.2% of 130 non-operated (p = 0.63).

There was a clear excess reporting among the patients with later cholecystectomy of having been advised to have an operation that was not done (Table 3). At first, this difference seems paradoxical in that one would expect relatively more of the non-operated patients to report a history of reluctance to undergo surgery. However, it is likely that some of the operated patients had already been advised to have their gallbladders removed by the time they completed the questionnaire and they were not yet willing to have that

Table 3. Attitudes toward medical care reported at multiphasic health checkups by gallstone patients with mild symptoms who did and did not later undergo cholecystectomy.

	Cholecystectomy		None		
	Total No. responding	% yes	Total No. responding	% yes	p
Changed doctors often?[a]	48	33.3	146	45.9	0.17
Satisfied with your medical care?[a]	30	70.0	97	68.0	0.84
Should doctors be able to cure eveything?	38	10.5	117	12.0	0.81
Ever advised to have an operation which was not done?	40	35.0	127	16.5	0.01
Should a person with a cold . . .	47		127		
see a doctor right away?		36.2		24.4	
treat himself unless it gets worse?		42.6		37.8	0.09
let nature take its course?		21.3		37.8	

[a] The reference period for the question was the year before the checkup.

particular operation. It is also possible that some of the non-operated patients were poor surgical risks and not advised to undergo cholecystectomy. These data are therefore difficult to interpret, but they at least do not indicate a frequent history of reluctance to have surgery among the non-operated group.

Another question reflecting attitude toward medical care showed an association with cholecystectomy which was of borderline significance (Table 3). Relatively more persons with later cholecystectomy believed that a person with a cold should see a doctor right away whereas persons who did not receive the operation believed more often that a person with a cold should let nature take its course. If one views the three possible responses to this question as a gradient between therapeutic activism and therapeutic nihilism, a Mantel-Haensel chi-square test for trend is appropriate and was statistically significant (p = 0.03).

No significant differences between the gallstone patients with and without subsequent cholecystectomies were observed for responses to questions about having changed doctors often, satisfaction with their medical care, and belief that doctors should be able to cure everything (Table 3).

Discussion

Initially, this search for characteristics (other than symptoms) predictive of undergoing elective cholecystectomy appeared to be disappointing. Many characteristics studied showed little if any association with having the operation. We did find that patients with subsequent cholecystectomy were more often female and tended to be younger when gallstones were diagnosed. They were also more apt to smoke cigarettes but not to consume alcohol appreciably more. They showed no more or less self-reported worry or depression. Not surprisingly, responses to one question showed a more activist view about seeking medical care.

We tried to determine whether a combination of predictive characteristics could be used as an indicator of the likelihood of subsequent cholecystectomy. First, we tried to form a high- and low-likelihood group using four characteristics. The hypothesized high-likelihood group was composed of women below age 50 yr at time of diagnosis who smoked cigarettes and believed that a person with a cold should see a doctor right away. The hypothesized low-likelihood group consisted of men age 50 yr and over who did not smoke and believed that a person with a cold should let nature take its course. Unfortunately, these groups contained only three (with one subsequent cholecystectomy) and six (with no subsequent cholecystectomies) persons, respectively, and could not be expected to provide reliable findings. A second approach was to focus on only two characteristics, sex and the answer to the question about treatment of a cold. Women who advocated seeing a doctor right away proved to have a much higher probability of cholecystectomy than men who believed in letting nature take its course, and the remaining subjects were intermediate (Table 4); probability (p) values for this analysis were 0.02 using an ordinary chi-square test and 0.01 using a chi-square test for trend.

These pilot data suggest that with more intensive studies of this type it may be possible to develop a fairly accurate profile of persons likely and unlikely to undergo elective cholecystectomy for gallstones, if it is recommended. This information could be of use in planning the management and follow-up of individual patients. For example, if it is important that a

Table 4. Ability of two characteristics to predict subsequent elective cholecystectomy in patients with mildly symptomatic gallstones.

Predicted likelihood of cholecystectomy[a]	Total No. of patients with mildly symptomatic gallstones	Subsequent cholecystectomy	
		No.	%
High	35	13	37.1
Medium	145	35	24.1
Low	14	0	0.0

[a] High-likelihood: women who believe that a person with a cold should see a doctor right away. Low-likelihood: men who believe that a person with a cold should let nature take its course. Medium-likelihood: everybody else.

particular patient in a low-likelihood group receive the operation or that one in a high-likelihood group not receive it, special counseling may be indicated. Information about characterisics associated with elective cholecystectomy is also valuable in comparing the outcomes of surgical vs. medical management. For example, if cigarette smoking is confirmed to be associated with elective cholecystectomy, then comparisons of mortality following these two approaches will have to take into account the deleterious effects of smoking.

Acknowledgments

This study was supported by Grant #R35 CA 49761 from the National Cancer Institute. Bruce Folck carried out the computer programming.

References

1. Bateson MC (1984): Gallbladder disease and cholecystectomy rate are independently variable. *Lancet* 2: 621—4.
2. Office of Disease Prevention and Health Promotion (1988): *Disease Prevention/Health Promotion: The Facts*, pp. 289—98, Palo Alto, California: Bull Publishing Company.
3. Ransohoff DF, Gracie WA, Wolfenson LB, Neuhauser D (1983): Prophylactic cholecystectomy or expectant management for silent gallstones: a decision analysis to assess survival. *Ann Intern Med* 99: 199—204.
4. Fitzpatrick G, Neutra R, Gilbert JP (1977): Cost-effectiveness of cholecystectomy for silent gallstones, pp. 246—61 in: Bunker JP, Barnes BA, Mosteller F (eds), *Cost, Risks and Benefits of Surgery*, New York, Oxford University Press.
5. Kottke TE, Feldman RD, Albert DA (1984): The risk ratio is insufficient for clinical decisions: the case of prophylactic cholecystectomy. *Med Decis Making* 4: 177—94.
6. Friedman GD, Raviola CA, Fireman B (1989): Prognosis of gallstones with mild or no symptoms: 25 years of follow-up in a health maintenance organization. *J Clin Epidemiol* 42: 127—36.
7. Collen MF, Davis LF (1969): The multitest laboratory in health care. *J Occup Med* 11: 355—60.

PART THREE

Risk factor for gallstone disease

11. Prevalence of gallstone disease in thalassaemia minor

V. ALVISI, P. PAZZI and D. SIGHINOLFI

There is much evidence to support the association between pigmentary cholelithiasis and chronic haemolytic anaemias [1—5], including prosthetic heart valve-induced haemolysis [6]. In this which is a former malaria district over 10% of the population is formed by heterozygotes with β-thalassaemia trait. However, this being a condition which is found all over the world, it is possible to calculate that there are no fewer than 5 million carriers of the thalassaemic trait in the Mediterranean area alone [7].

This condition is associated with continuous, low-grade haemolysis [8, 9]: the excessive production of bilirubin due to haemolysis, therefore represents an important prerequisite for the formation of pigment gallstones. Furthermore, it has been observed that the mean serum level of total cholesterol is significantly lower in carriers of thalassaemic trait as compared to normal homozygotes [10, 11]; there are also suggestions in the literature that the β-thalassaemia trait may protect against cardiovascolar disease [12]. The possible interrelation between gallstone disease, cholesterol metabolism and atherosclerosis, represents yet another point of interest in the thalassaemic population.

The aim of our study was to determine the real prevalence of gallstone disease in subjects with thalassaemia minor compared with normal homozygotes, in order to identify which individual and biochemical features are associated with the presence of gallstones.

Materials and methods

Two separate studies were carried out. The first study was part of a wide cross-sectional Italian multicentre survey on gallbladder disease in a free-living population (MICOL). The resident population of Codigoro was studied; a small town situated in an area which had, in the past, a high incidence of malaria. From the electoral list a selection was made of the subjects aged between 29 and 69 yr: of the 3691 subjects selected, 2510 (68%) took part in the study. The protocol consisted mainly of: an ultrason-

L. Capocaccia et al. (eds), Recent advances in the epidemiology and prevention of gallstone disease, 73—81.
© 1991 *Kluwer Academic Publishers. Printed in the Netherlands.*

ographic examination of the abdomen; a standard questionnaire (including demographic and social data, medical and family history and dietary habits); measures of height and weight; a set of blood tests, including determination of red blood cell indices. In the presence of values of mean corpuscolar volume (MCV) $< 79\,\mu^3$ and mean corpuscolar haemoglobin (MCH) $<$ 27 pg we proceeded to electrophoresis of haemoglobin, the diagnosis of β-thalassaemia heterozygote being confirmed by values of $HbA_2 > 3.5\%$. The second study involved a selected population of patients admitted to a Department of Internal Medicine for various medical pathologies. The studies consisted of 1043 patients, consecutively hospitalized, who underwent routine untrasonographic examination of the upper abdomen regardless of the nature of the disease for which they were admitted. The carriers of β-thalassaemic trait were also identified in this study on the basis of low MCV, low MCH and increased HbA_2.

Results

The epidemiological study of the Codigoro population revealed 317 carriers of heterozygote thalassaemia (12.6% of the total sample). The data concerning the prevalence of gallstones, previous cholecystectomy and gallstone disease (gallstone + cholecystectomy), reported in Table 1, evidenced a higher prevalence of gallstone disease in thalassaemic patients, even though the difference was not statistically significant. By analysing the data separately, with regard to sex, it was observed that the prevalence of cholecystectomy and total gallbladder disease in non-thalassaemic subjects was significantly higher in females, whereas no such significant difference between the sexes was present in the group of 317 thalassaemics. The difference in prevalence of gallstone disease between the two groups considered was particularly evident in the lower age group but was inverted in the over-sixties (Fig. 1). In a comparison of the patients with gallstones, the two groups were found to be homogeneous as far as mean age and body

Table 1. Prevalence of gallstone disease (gallstones + cholecystectomy in the epidemiological study (2510 subjects).

	Epidemiological study (2510 subjects)	
	Thalassaemic carriers (n = 317)	Controls (n = 2193)
Age (yr)	50.1 ± 10.8	50.2 ± 10.7
Gallstones	31 (9.8%)	166 (7.5%)
Cholecystectomy	23 (7.8%)	153 (7.0%)
Gallstones-disease	54 (17.0%)	319 (14.5%)

Table 2. Prevalence of gallstone disease by sex in the epidemiological study.

	Males		Females	
	Thalass. (n = 145)	Controls (n = 1071)	Thalass. (n = 172)	Controls (n = 1122)
Gallstones	13 (9.0%)	80 (7.5%)	18 (10.5%)	86 (7.7%)
Cholecystectomy	6 (4.1%)	45 (4.2%)	17 (9.9%)	108 (9.6%)[a]
Gallbladder-disease	19 (13.1%)	125 (11.7%)	35 (20.4%)	194 (17.3%)[a]

[a] Males versus females p < 0.001 only in control group.

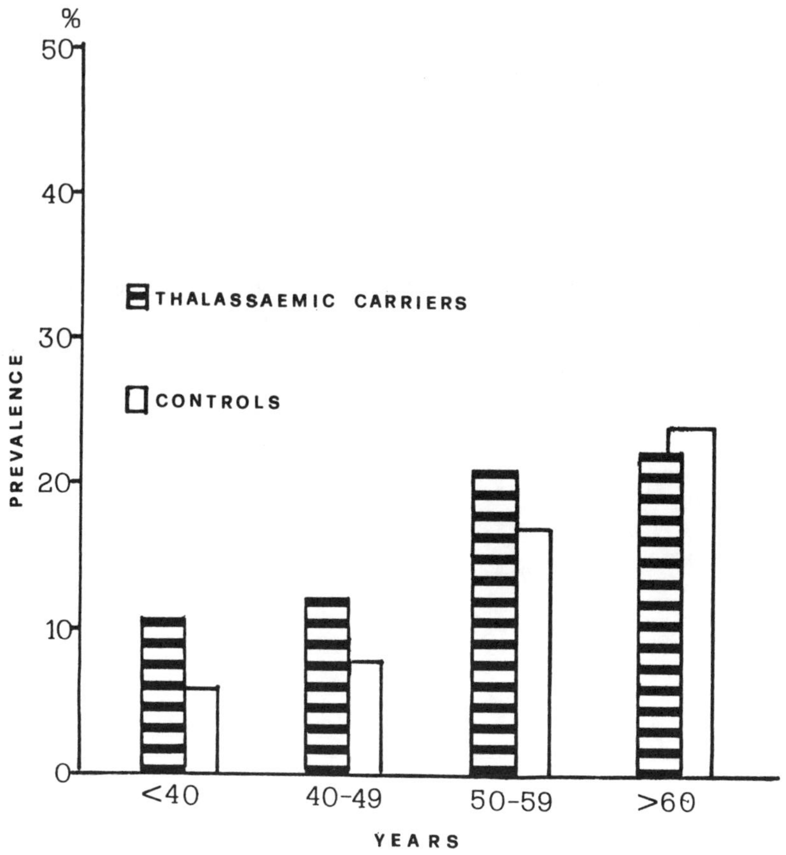

Fig. 1. Prevalence of gallstone disease (gallstones + cholecystectomy) in 2510 subjects, divided by age group.

mass index were concerned, whereas comparison of some biochemical data revealed a significantly higher level of total cholesterol and blood glucose in the 166 non-thalassaemic subjects with gallstone disease (Table 3). Since it is well known that thalassaemics present a lower packed-cell volume (PCV) than normal subjects, we adjusted the values obtained for PCV complement, i.e. the plasma volume percentage, thus making the serum concentrations more comparable. Comparison of the adjusted data did not reveal any significant differeces among the parameters examined and in particular the difference observed regarding total cholesterol (adjusted data: 116.1 ± 20.8 mg dl⁻¹ in thalassaemics versus 120.9 ± 21.7 mg dl) and blood glucose (52.4 ± 4.9 mg dl⁻¹ versus 55.5 ± 8.4 mg dl⁻¹ respectively) disappeared. The data concerning hospitalized patients (Table 4) also evidenced a higher prevalence of gallstone disease in the 106 carriers of β-thalassaemia trait: a markedly increased overall frequency of cholecystectomy (18.9%) was observed. The increased prevalence of disease in this population was interpreted on the basis of two considerations: on the one hand, the population was a selected one in that it was chosen from subjects hospitalized for various medical conditions, and the other hand it was made up of subjects at an advanced age (mean age over 60 yr), in which gallstone disease is known to reach its highest frequency. For this population, too, the marked difference

Table 3. Some clinical and biochemical data of gallstone patients of the epidemiological study.

	Thalass. (31)	Controls (166)
Age (yr)	53.4 ± 9.2	55.6 ± 9.3
BMI (kg m⁻²)	26.1 ± 3.2	26.9 ± 7.3
HDL-Cholest. (mg dl⁻¹)	55.7 ± 15.7	56.7 ± 14.5
Total Cholest. (mg dl⁻¹)	190.3 ± 33.8	217.7 ± 43.3[a]
Triglycerides (mg dl⁻¹)	101.1 ± 51.5	109.7 ± 98.8
Blood Glucose (mg dl⁻¹)	86.1 ± 8.6	92.3 ± 15.6[b]

[a] $p < 0.01$.
[b] $p < 0.05$.

Table 4. Prevalence of gallstone disease among 1043 hospitalized patients.

	Thalassaemic carriers (n = 106)	Controls (n = 937)
Age (yr)	61.2 ± 14.5	62.7 ± 15.0
Gallstones	24 (22.6%)	211 (22.5%)
Cholecystectomy	20 (18.9%)	125 (13.3%)
Gallstone-disease	44 (41.5%)	336 (35.8%)

in the prevalence of total gallstone disease and cholecystectomy between males and females was only observed in subjects who were not carriers of the thalassaemic trait (Table 5). Once again, the blood level of total cholesterol (Table 6) was significantly lower in subjects with gallstones and β-thalassaemia trait compared to non thalassaemic gallstone subjects; in this case, too, adjustment of cholesterol values for PCV did not reveal any substantial difference. In this population of hospitalized patients we observed a progressive increase in the prevalence of gallstone disease in relation to age, but in all age groups the prevalence was higher in thalassaemic carriers: the difference in prevalence between the two groups was however significant only in the under 50 age groups (Fig. 2). As far as the presence of clinical symptoms was concerned, among the hospitalized patients, only 3 out of the 24 thalassaemic patients with gallstone disease (13%) had at least one episode of a typical biliary colic in the 5 yr preceding the study, compared to 67 out of the 144 (32%) gallstone non-thalassaemic subjects. Moreover, only 17% of the thalassaemics knew they had gallstones, compared to 44% of non-thalassaemics ($X^2 = 5.403$, $p = 0.02$). The presence of typical biliary colic presented, in thalassaemic subjects, a characteristic trend in relation to age, both in hospitalized gallstone subjects and in those participating in the epidemiological study. In fact, gallstone disease was more frequently symptomatic in younger subjects. This trend was found to be statistically significant

Table 5. Prevalence of gallstone disease by sex in 1043 hospitalized patients.

	Males		Females	
	Thalass. (n = 35)	Controls (n = 319)	Thalass. (n = 71)	Controls (n = 618)
Gallstones	9 (25.7%)	63 (19.7%)	15 (21.1%)	148 (23.9%)
Cholecystectomy	3 (8.6%)	19 (6.0%)	17 (23.9%)	106 (17.2%)[a]
Gallstone-disease	12 (34.3%)	82 (25.7%)	32 (45.0%)	245 (41.1%)[a]

[a] Males versus females p < 0.001 only in control group.

Table 6. Some clinical and biochemical data of gallstone hospital patients.

	Thalassaemic carriers (n = 24)	Controls (n = 211)
Age (yr)	70.6 ± 10.6	68.9 ± 11.7
R.B.W. (%)	122.1 ± 28.1	116.2 ± 20.5
Cholesterol (mg dl^{-1})	182.0 ± 60.6	203.5 ± 56.4[a]
Triglycerides (mg dl^{-1})	106.9 ± 43.5	129.4 ± 86.0
Blood Glucose (mg dl^{-1})	113.6 ± 38.8	128.4 ± 62.9

[a] p < 0.05.

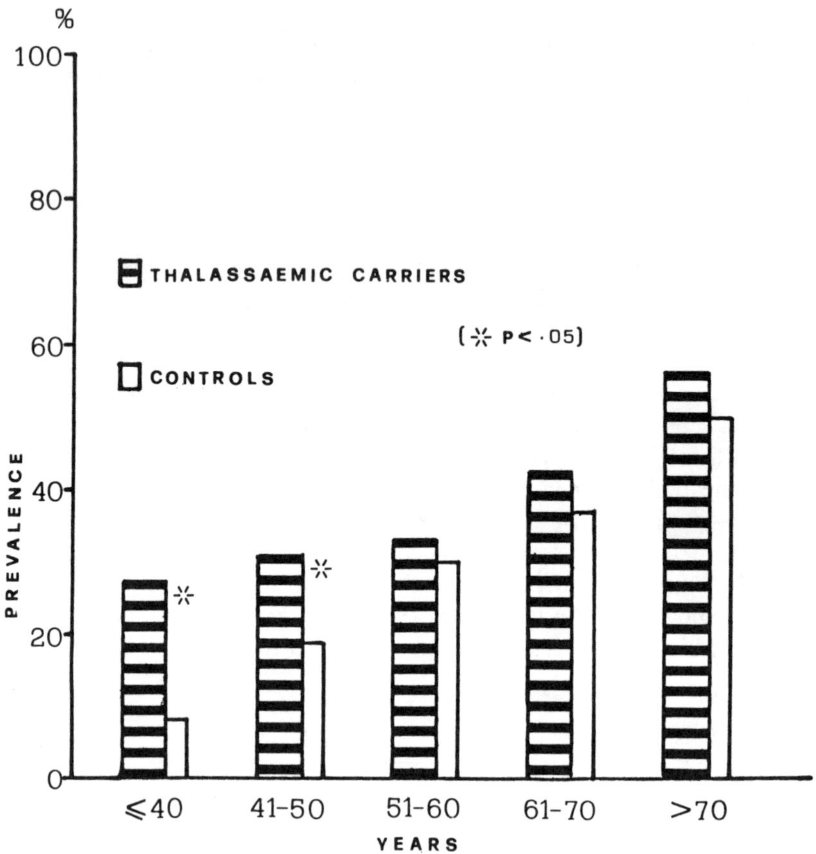

Fig. 2. Prevalence of gallstone disease (gallstones + cholecystectomy) in 1043 consecutive hospital patients, divided by age group.

in the thalassaemic gallstone subjects included in the epidemiological study (Fig. 3), whereas it was not so in non-thalassaemic gallstone subjects. No significant difference was observed, however, between the two groups regarding the number and size of gallstones, even if, in thalassaemics, gallstones were more frequently multiple (71% versus 56%) and smaller than 15 mm (71% versus 63%), just as the characteristics of the gallstones did not seem to be related to the presence of biliary pain.

Discussion

In two separate studies regarding a free-living population and an in-patient one, we encountered a tendentially higher prevalence of gallstone disease in β-thalassaemic trait carriers than in subjects comparable for ethnic back-

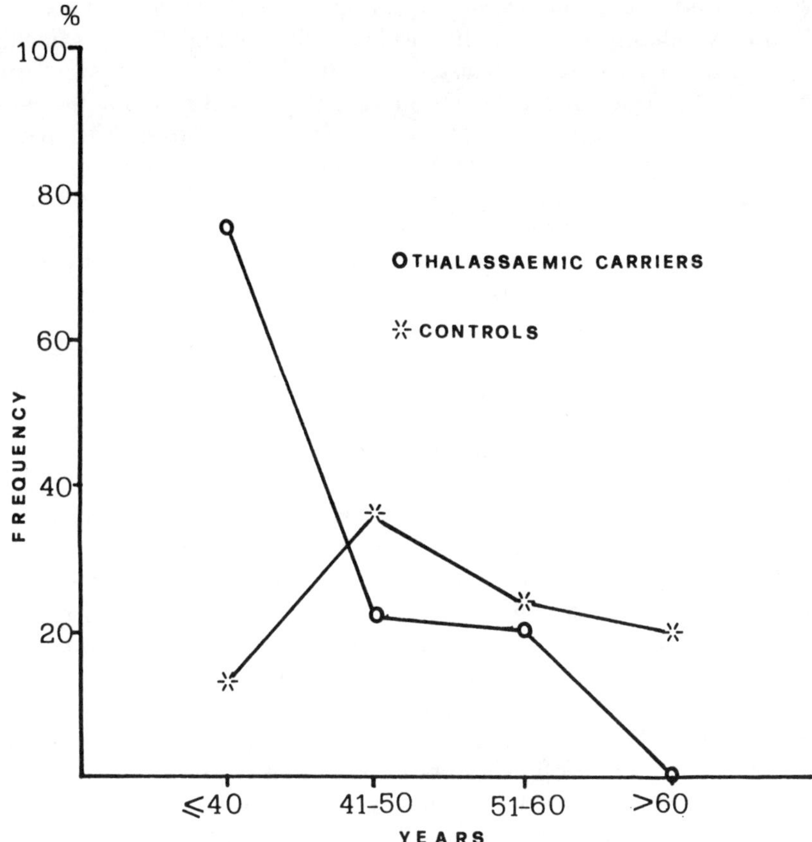

Fig. 3. Frequency of biliary colic in gallstone patients (in thalassaemic carriers $X^2 = 8.405$, $p < 0.05$).

ground, dietary habits and no known haemolytic anaemias. In a previous untrasonographic study on 84 females with thalassaemia minor, a higher prevalence of cholelithiasis, as compared to controls, was reported [13], and in a series of 128 individuals, heterozygous for β-thalassaemia, 22 had gallstone related symptoms [14]. However, rather than prevalence of gallstone disease in absolute terms several considerations may be made on the basis of our results: *firstly*, the strong correlation between the female sex and gallstone disease found in the control population, was not observed in the group of thalassaemics we studied. This finding obviously brings to mind the analagous epidemiological distributions, characteristic of pigment gallstones, which, unlike that of cholesterol stones, is equally distributed between the two sexes [15, 16].

Secondly, the presence of β-thalassaemic trait would seem to affect the presence of gallstone disease particularly in younger age groups. Given the lack of up-to-date data on the type of gallstones present in these subjects, we can only hypothesize that this chronic haemolitic condition may somehow accelerate the appearance of gallstones in metabolically 'predisposed' subjects. As for the lower frequency of symptomatic cases observed in thalassaemics, one must bear in mind (at least as far as our hospitalized patient population is concerned) the role that the increased cholecystectomy level may have played in selection of previously symptomatic cases. Furthermore, this interpretation would seem to be partially supported by the observation that the symptomatic cases in the thalassaemics were more frequently encountered in younger subjects.

Thirdly, in the thalassaemic subjects we generally observed a hypocholesterolaemia, or at least a mean level of cholesterolaemia, which was lower than that of normal homozygotes. Since we were dealing with anaemic subjects they presented MCV and PCV values below normal range. It is well-known that a significant correlation exists between haemoglobin level and serum levels of cholesterol [17, 18] which is most likely linked to the variation in plasma volume. The reduced levels we observed in cholesterolaemia would seem to be related to diluition of the same pool of circulating cholesterol in a higher plasmatic volume. In fact, when the cholesterol concentration was adjusted no substantial difference was observed between thalassaemics and non-thalassaemics. Previous epidemiological studies [19] have demonstrated a negative association between the presence of gallstones and total serum cholesterol concentration. A low level of total cholesterolaemia observed in thalassaemic subjects may, therefore, be considered a further possible risk factor for gallstone development.

Since the method used in our studies to identify gallstone disease was ultrasonographic examination we have no information on the type of stone encountered. Above all, we do not know if pigmentary gallstone disease which is known to be associated with a chronic haemolytic condition, is in fact more frequent in β-thalassaemic carriers. To this regard, future studies on appropriate sample groups of gallstone subjects should employ methodologies which are suitably sensitive to and specific for identification of the chemical composition of the gallstones. One such study could be a microscopic examination of crystals in duodenal bile.

References

1. Jordan RA (1957): Cholelithiasis in sickle cell disease. *Gastroenterology* 33: 952—58.
2. Cameron JL, Maddrey WC, Zuidema GD (1971): Biliary tract disease in sickle cell anemia: surgical considerations. *Ann Surg* 174: 702—10.
3. Bates GC, Braun CH (1952): Incidence of gallbladder disease in chronic hemolytic anemia (spherocytosis). *Gastroenterology* 21: 104—109.
4. Dewey KW, Grossman H, Canale VC (1970): Cholelithiasis in thalassemia major. *Radiology* 96: 385—88.

5. Pappis CH, Galanakis S, Moussatos G (1989): Experience of splenectomy and cholecystectomy in children with chronic haemolytic anaemia. *J Pediatr Surg* 24: 543—46.
6. Merendino KA, Manhas DR (1973): Man-made gallstones: a new entity following cardiac valve replacement. *Ann Surg* 177: 694—704.
7. Weatherall DJ, Clegg JB (1981): *The thalassemia syndromes*. Oxford, Blackwell Scientific Publications.
8. Gallo E, Pich P, Ricco G, Saglio G, Camaschella C, Mazza U (1975): The relationships between anemia, fecal stercobilinogen, erythrocyte survival, and globin synthesis in heterozygotes for β-thalassemia. *Blood* 46: 693—99.
9. Cazzola M, Alessandrino P, Barosi G, Morandi S, Stefanelli M (1979): Quantitative evaluation of the mechanisms of the anaemia in heterozygous β-thalassaemia. *Scand J Haematol* 23: 107—111.
10. Fessas P, Stamatoyannopoulos G, Keys A (1963): Serum Cholesterol and thalassaemia trait. *Lancet* 1: 1182–3.
11. Malamos B, Fessas P, Stamatoyannopoulos G (1962): Types of thalassaemia-trait carriers as revealed by a study of their incidence in Greece. *Brit J Hematol* 8: 5—11.
12. Crowley JP, Sheth S, Capone RJ, Schilling RF (1987): A paucity of thalassemia trait in Italian men with myocardial infarction. *Acta Haematol* 78: 249—51.
13. Borgna-Pignatti C, De Stefano P, Bongo IG, Tomasi G, Gatti C (1983): Cholelithiasis in thalassaemia minor: a prevalence study in Italian women. *Ital J Gastroenterol* 15: 228—30.
14. Gardikass C (1968): Modes of presentation of thalassemia minor. *Acta Haematol* 40: 34—42.
15. Trotman BW, Soloway RD (1975): Pigment vs cholesterol cholelithiasis: clinical and epidemiological aspects. *Am J Dig Dis* 20: 735—40.
16. Miyake H, Johnston CG (1968): Gallstones: ethnological studies. *Digestion* 1: 219—28.
17. Elwood PC, Mahler R, Sweetnam P, Moore F, Welsby E (1970): Association between circulating haemoglobin level, serum cholesterol and blood pressure. *Lancet* 1: 589—90.
18. Böttiger LE, Carlson LA (1972): Relation between serum cholesterol and triglyceride concentration and haemoglobin values in non-anaemic healthy persons. *Br Med J* 3: 731.
19. Angelico M, GREPCO Group (1984): In: Capocaccia L, Ricci G, Angelico F, Angelico M, Attili AF (eds.), *Epidemiology and Prevention of Gallstone Disease*, pp. 77—84, Lancaster, MTP Press.

12. Cholelithiasis and blood groups: evidence for a lack of association

A. DE SANTIS, S. GINANNI CORRADINI, E. P. GIULIANI, A. F. ATTILI and THE OPERATIVE UNIT OF ROMA I OF THE MICOL GROUP

It is a widely held view that there is a close association between certain diseases of the digestive tract and blood groups. A significant statistical correlation has been shown between duodenal ulcers and blood group 0 [1] and between gastric cancer and blood group A [2]. Possible links between cholelithiasis and blood groups in the ABO system have been studied in the past. Unfortunately, the data published often disagree. Some authors found a positive association between biliary gallstones and blood group AB [3], while others found that this was associated with group A [4—7]. Some authors failed to find any association between lithiasis of the gallbladder and ABO blood groups [8, 9]. Moreover, a negative association was sometimes found between this disease and specific blood groups such as B [3], 0 [6, 7] and the Rh factor [10]. None of these studies were performed on a free-living population or had used homogeneous control groups and, in the majority of cases, gallstone diagnosis was only obtained clinically. Thus, any possible association between cholelithiasis and blood group has not been proven. On the other hand, this issue would appear to be of interest in that the genes which codify for antigenes of the ABO and Rh systems could play the role of genetic marker of this disease, assuming that cholelithiasis develops where there is a genetic predisposition determined by the presence of one or more anomalous genes.

This study looked at the correlation between ABO and Rh blood groups and biliary gallstones during a recent epidemiological survey on a free-living population sample [11]. All participants were submitted to an ultrasonographic examination of the gallbladder and biliary tree in order to diagnose the presence or not of gallstones.

Materials and methods

The study was performed on a free-living population sample between July 1985 and July 1986. 2615 individuals randomly sampled from the electoral list of Tivoli, a small town near Rome, were examined during an epidemiological screening for gallstone disease as part of the Multicenter Italian study on Epidemiology of Cholelithiasis (MICOL) [11].

For all participants:

(1) a fasting blood sample to determine total cholesterol, HDL cholesterol, triglycerides and glucose was taken;

(2) an ultrasonography of the gallbladder and biliary tree using a Kontron, Mod Sigma 20, equipped with a 3.5 MHz linear transducer, was performed;

(3) height and weight were measured;

(4) a questionnaire was completed (data are not reported here).

ABO blood group and the Rh factor were determined in the first 1625 individuals examined (62.1%). The test was made on a blood sample taken by venopuncture using a standard slide method.

Of the 1625 individuals examined, 776 (47.8%) were males and 849 (52.2%) females, with an average age of 48.9 $\pm$ 11.8 yr (range 20—69 yr).

Data were processed using a PC statistics package. Student's t-test for unpaired data and the Chi-square were used to assess, respectively, the differences between the means and frequencies observed. A probability level equal to or above 5% was accepted as being significant.

Results

Table 1 shows the prevalence of cholelithiasis, cholecystectomy and gallbladder disease (cholelithiasis + cholecystectomy) in ABO and Rh blood groups. No statistical difference arose regarding the prevalence of cholelithiasis, cholecystectomy or gallbladder disease in individuals with different blood groups with the exception of a higher frequency of cholecystectomy in the Rh negative group (p = 0.029).

Table 1. Prevalence of cholelithiasis, cholecystectomy or gallbladder disease (cholelithiasis + cholecystectomy) in ABO and Rh blood groups.

	Normals		Cholelithiasis		Cholecystectomy		Gallbladder disease	
	n	%	n	%	n	%	n	%
A	479	77	78	12.5	65	10.5	143	23
B	160	80.4	23	11.5	16	8.1	39	19.6
AB	46	70.8	12	18.5	7	10.7	19	29.2
0	556	75.3	90	12.2	93	12.5	183	24.7
Rh +	1030	77	170	12.7	138	10.3	308	23
Rh −	211	73.5	33	11.5	43	15[a]	76	26.5

[a] p = 0.029.

Tables 2 and 3 show the mean values of certain variables commonly considered to be associated with cholelithiasis in participants divided according to their blood group. Respect to all the other blood group subjects, serum cholesterol levels were significantly higher amongst blood groups A and Rh positive ($p < 0.01$ and $p = 0.021$, respectively). Moreover, the latter also had significantly higher triglyceride levels ($p = 0.001$). No differences were found in the values of the other variables measured. Sex distribution and parity were similar in the different blood groups. Since the above differences might have affected the prevalence of GD in the various blood groups, a multivariate analysis was performed in which the presence of gallbladder

Table 2. Mean values ± SD or ratio of certain variables commonly considered to be associated with cholelithiasis in ABO blood groups.

	Blood groups			
	A	B	AB	O
Age (yr)	49.2 ± 11.9	48.3 ± 11.9	47.9 ± 10.6	48.9 ± 11.8
Triglycerides[a]	150.3 ± 104.9	144.2 ± 88.9	151.2 ± 123.1	146.5 ± 91.5
Cholesterol[a]	230.9 ± 44.8[b]	215.4 ± 44.6	216.8 ± 42.7	226.2 ± 46.6
HDL cholesterol[a]	52.3 ± 14.1	52.3 ± 13.7	49.2 ± 13.4	52.2 ± 13.3
Glucose[a]	91.1 ± 20.8	92.5 ± 26.3	88.7 ± 13.9	90.7 ± 19.1
BMI	27.6 ± 4.2	27.4 ± 4.4	28.4 ± 4.6	27.5 ± 4.2
Parity (n)	2.0 ± 4.0	2.2 ± 1.2	1.9 ± 1.0	2.1 ± 1.2
Men/women	0.9	0.9	1.1	0.9

[a] Values expressed in mg dL^{-1}.
[b] $p < 0.01$ A versus B, A versus AB, A versus others.

Table 3. Mean values ± SD or ratio of certain variables commonly considered to be associated with cholelithiasis in Rhesus blood groups.

	Rh +	Rh −
Age (yr)	48.9 ± 11.7	48.8 ± 12.3
Triglycerides[a]	149.9 ± 100.4[b]	138.4 ± 84.5
Cholesterol[a]	227.2 ± 46.2[c]	222.1 ± 43.6
HDL cholesterol[a]	51.9 ± 13.6	53.2 ± 13.8
Glucose[a]	90.9 ± 20.8	91.4 ± 19.6
BMI	27.6 ± 4.3	27.2 ± 3.9
Parity (n)	2.1 ± 1.2	2.2 ± 1.2
Men/women	0.9	0.9

[a] Values expressed in mg dL^{-1}.
[b] $p = 0.001$.
[c] $p = 0.021$.

disease was taken as a dependent variable and cholesterol, HDL cholesterol, triglycerides, glucose, age, sex, BMI (Body Mass Index), parity and blood groups were considered as predictive variables. The final equation did not show any significant association between the blood groups examined and gallbladder disease.

Discussion

This study shows that no significant association exists between gallbladder disease and blood groups. This finding is in contradiction with most existing studies on this topic [3—7, 10]. However, these only observed cases where gallbladder disease was clinically evident. Recent epidemiological studies have clearly shown that only a minority of the subjects with gallstones are aware of having gallstones or are symptomatic [12, 13]. The main weakness of the previous studies on the association between gallbladder disease and blood groups is the poor definition of the endpoint. In addition, the control populations were mostly composed of blood donors from blood transfusion centres [3—6, 9, 10]. This could cause a bias due to the major prevalence of 0 and AB blood groups in these populations [7]. A comparison between the distribution of blood groups in the population studied here and those of the blood transfusion centre at Tivoli confirms this finding. Those with blood group O were 45.5% of the population sample studied versus 51.5% of blood donors at the centre (p < 0.05).

In our study, the univariate analysis showed a higher frequency of cholecystectomies in Rh negative subjects which, however, disappeared at multivariate analysis. This indicates that this association is not independent of other variables (age, sex, BMI, triglycerides, cholesterol, glucose). Similar results were found by Bodvall and Overgaard [7] who failed to find any association between cholecystectomy and the Rh factor. The univariate analysis showed significantly higher blood cholesterol levels in blood groups A and Rh positive. Moreover, the latter also showed significantly higher triglyceride levels than Rh negative subjects. An association between blood cholesterol levels and of belonging to blood group A has been described elsewhere [14, 15]. As both cholesterol and triglycerides have been described as being associated with cholelithiasis [16], in order to reveal possible associations, hidden by the effect of certain correlated variables, a multivariate analysis was performed. No significant relationship emerged between ABO and Rh blood groups and cholelithiasis. This finding is not surprising because the contradictory conclusions of the previous studies are probably owing to mere chance for the lack of any true association between blood groups and cholelithiasis.

Finally, from our study and from a review of the previous studies, it can be concluded that belonging to a specific blood group does not increase the risk of gallstone disease nor can this be used as a genetic marker.

References

1. Langman MJS, Doll R, Scaracci R (1967): ABO blood group and secretor status in stomal ulcer. *Gut* 8: 128—132.
2. Aird I, Bentall HH, Roberts JAF (1953): A relationship between cancer of the stomach and the ABO blood groups. *Brit Med J* 1: 799—801.
3. Hauch EW, Moore FJ (1963): Is cholelithiasis associated with a specific blood group? *Gastroenterology* 44: 125—126.
4. Massa G, Gnavi M, Baggi G, Scevola G (1980): Sull'associazione tra colelitiasi e gruppi sanguigni ABO. *Minerva Medica* 71: 2993—2995.
5. Chakravartti MR, Chakravartti R (1979): ABO blood groups in cholelithiasis. *Ann Génét* 22: 171—172.
6. Lindskog BI (1973): Association between the ABO blood group and stone in the deep bile ducts. *Acta Chir Scand* 139: 270—272.
7. Bodvall B, Overgaard B (1966): The association between ABO blood groups and cholelithiasis with special reference to biliary distress following cholecystectomy. *Acta Chir Scand* 131: 334—342.
8. Lisker R, Mutchinik ORZ, de las Fuentas G (1981): Falta de asociation entre los grupos sanguineos del sistema ABO y la colelitiasis. *Rev Invest Clin* 33: 269—272.
9. Monaci R, Meoni S, Bini D, Morganti G (1984): Associazione gruppi sanguigni ABO e calcolosi della colecisti: un'opinione contraria. *Minerva Medica* 75: 2221—2226.
10. Orlando R, Piccoli A, Riz G, Naccarato R, Okolicsanyi L (1981): Associazione tra gruppi sanguigni ABO, colelitiasi e sindrome di Gilbert. *Minerva dietologica e gastroenterologica* 27: 47—50.
11. Multicentrica Italiana Colelitiasi (MICOL) (1988): Reliability study on ultrasonographic detection of gallstones: The MICOL experience, in: *Pathochemistry, Pathophysiology and Pathomechanics of the Biliary System. New Strategies for the Treatment of Biliary Tract Disease*, Abstract Book, 131.
12. Gruppo Romano per la Epidemiologia e la Prevenzione della Colelitiasi (GREPCO) (1984): Prevalence of gallstone disease in an Italian adult female population. *Am J Epidemiol* 119: 796—805.
13. Gruppo Romano per la Epidemiologia e la Prevenzione della Colelitiasi (GREPCO) (1988): The epidemiology of gallstone disease in Rome, Italy. Part 1. Prevalence data in men *Hepatology* 8: 904—906.
14. Oliver MF, Geizerova H, Cumming RA, Heady JA (1969): Serum cholesterol and ABO and Rhesus blood groups *Lancet* Sept. 605—606.
15. Langman MJS, Elwood PC, Foote J, Ryrie DR (1969): ABO and Lewis blood groups and serum cholesterol. *Lancet* Sept. 607—609.
16. Gruppo Romano per la Epidemiologia e la Prevenzione della Colelitiasi (GREPCO) (1988): The epidemiology of gallstone disease in Rome, Italy. Part II. Factors associated with the disease. *Hepatology* 8: 904—906.

13. Genetic, ethnic, and environmental factors: findings from the San Antonio heart study

A. K. DIEHL

As discussed in Chapter 4 of this volume, recent studies indicate that Mexican Americans have a prevalence of gallstones that is 1.5 to 2 times that of non-Hispanic whites. The factors underlying the higher rates in this ethnic group remain to be fully explored. Nevertheless, four possible explanations can be offered.

First, the measured prevalences may be in error as a result of ascertainment bias. No study to date has determined the true prevalence of gallstone disease in population-based concurrent samples of Mexican Americans and non-Hispanic whites. The studies of Diehl et al., Hanis et al., and Samet et al. reported the prevalence of cholecystectomy or clinical diagnosis of gallstone disease [1—4]. Even assuming that the data obtained by these methods have substantial validity, true prevalences of gallstones are underestimated because many persons harboring stones remain asymptomatic and go undiagnosed. The extent of undercounting of cases is uncertain, but it is possible that the true rates may be twice or more those reported in these papers. Arevalo et al. have reported gallstone prevalences in concurrent samples of Latinos and other ethnic groups [5]. However, their data are derived from records of autopsies performed by the San Francisco County Coroner, and the prevalences reported may not reflect those of the general population. Maurer et al. have provided the only population-based prevalences based on cholecystectomy history and screening ultrasonography [6]. While their prevalence estimates for Mexican Americans are probably the best available, their methods did not include a concurrent sample of non-Hispanic whites.

The studies from San Antonio, Texas are in fact the only ones to concurrently examine Mexican Americans and non-Hispanic whites [1, 2]. Nevertheless, ethnicity-related variations in diagnostic practices might account for apparent differences in the prevalence of 'clinical' gallbladder disease. If, for example, physicians in San Antonio more readily order gallbladder ultrasonography for Mexican American patients with nonspecific abdominal symptoms, the detection of asymptomatic stones will be greater for Mexican Americans than for non-Hispanics, and the prevalences of clinically recognized galbladder disease will be biased. While we cannot disprove the existence of such a bias, there are no empirical data to support it, and we feel it is an unlikely explanation for our findings [2]. In addition, the Hispanic HANES prevalences have been compared to those determined during ultrasound studies in Denmark and Italy, and support the finding of an increased prevalence in Mexican American women [6]. Finally, gallbladder cancer mortality data also document gallbladder disease rates that are greater in Mexican Americans than non-Hispanic whites [7]. Overall, these studies indicate that the prevalence differences observed are not simply the result of biased ascertainment.

Although the ethnic differences in prevalence may be unbiased, they may still be confounded by widely accepted risk factors for gallstone disease. Body mass index, body fat distribution, parity, estrogen use, and other factors are related to gallstone risk and may vary substantially among ethnic populations in the United States. In fact, Mexican Americans of both sexes in the San Antonio heart study have a higher mean body mass index than non-Hispanic whites (both $p < 0.001$), and Mexican American women have higher mean parity ($p < 0.001$). Such potential confounding has been examined in a series of statistical analyses. We have found in a discriminant analysis that the prevalence of clinical gallbladder disease is greater in Mexican American women ($p = 0.05$) after age, body mass index, and parity are forced into the function. Other publications from this study have found that the higher prevalence in Mexican Americans remains statistically significant after adjustments for age, body mass index, body fat distribution, nutrient intake, and diabetes in logistic regression analyses [8—10]. Hence, confounding by recognized risk factors fails to explain the higher prevalence of gallbladder disease observed in Mexican Americans.

A third explanation for the ethnic difference, and the one we favor, is that the high prevalence of gallstones in Mexican Americans has a genetic basis. As discussed in Chapter 4, modern Mexican Americans reflect the admixture of Spaniards and other Europeans with Amerindians over a period of four centuries. We hypothesize that this Amerindian admixture accounts for their high rates of gallstone disease. The extraordinary prevalence of gallbladder disease in the Pima Indians of Arizona is widely recognized, but high rates of gallbladder disease have also been reported in Amerindian populations from Alaska, Canada, Minnesota, Oklahoma, New Mexico, and Bolivia [7]. These high rates are not limited to a few tribes, but appear to be common to Amerindian groups throughout North and South America despite their substantial differences in culture, environment, and diet. It is likely that these peoples share a genetically determined predisposition to gallstone formation. Studies employing genetic markers in Texas Mexican Americans estimate their Amerindian admixture to be 15 to 45% [11]. Hence, the prevalence of gallbladder disease in Mexican Americans — higher than that of non-Hispanic whites, but lower than that of full-blooded Amerindians — may have a genetic basis.

Three empirical observations support this hypothesis. First, Bolivian 'mestizos' have rates of gallbladder cancer which similarly fall between those of the Amerindian and European populations of that country [12]. Also, Hanis et al. have related gallbladder disease prevalence data from Starr County, Texas to individual admixture estimates determined from genetic markers. Their data support a relationship between Amerindian admixture and gallbladder disease prevalence, at least in women [11]. Finally, we have used an indirect measure of Amerindian admixture, skin reflectance, to examine this hypothesis in Mexican Americans from the San Antonio heart study [7]. Women in the darkest (most Amerindian) tertile had an age-standardized gallbladder disease prevalence of 21.0% versus 15.8% for those in the middle and 12.5% for those in the lightest (least Amerindian) tertile. Non-Hispanic white women had a prevalence of 8.7% [2]. Taken together, these data indicate that the high rates of gallbladder disease observed in Mexican Americans result from a genetic predisposition to stone formation introduced by their Amerindian ancestors.

A fourth possible explanation for Mexican Americans' high prevalence is confounding by poorly-established or unrecognized risk factors. Because in our community Mexican Americans are relatively disadvantaged in comparison to non-Hispanic whites, we examined socioeconomic status as a risk factor for clinical gallbladder disease [2]. Neighborhood of residence, educational attainment, occupational status, and family income served as measures of socioeconomic status. We found an inverse relationship of gallbladder disease prevalence to socioeconomic status in women of both ethnic groups (Fig. 1). Moreover, in logistic regression analyses in which age, body mass index, parity, and ethnic group were controlled for, we observed a 'dose-response' effect in that the risk of gallbladder disease rose with each decline in level of socioeconomic status. Interestingly, at high levels of socioeconomic status the ethnic differences in gallbladder disease prevalence narrowed or even reversed. Other reports from the San Antonio heart study document that Mexican Americans of high socioeconomic status have relatively little Amerindian admixture in comparison to Mexican Americans of low status [13].

Socioeconomic status in turn may be associated with a constellation of health habits (such as use of tobacco and alcohol), dietary preferences, biochemical values, medication use, and exposures which collectively can be considered 'environmental' in nature. That is, unlike many important risk factors for gallstones including age, gender, and genetic heritage, environmental factors are potentially modifiable, and may present opportunities for the prevention of gallstone disease.

We have subsequently examined several of these environmental factors. In a series of analyses, we found that frequency of alcohol use was inversely related to the prevalence of clinical gallbladder disease. Men who drank alcohol at least three times weekly had only one-third the risk of those who drank less than once a month, after adjustment for multiple potential confounders in a logistic regression analysis. We found a slightly increased

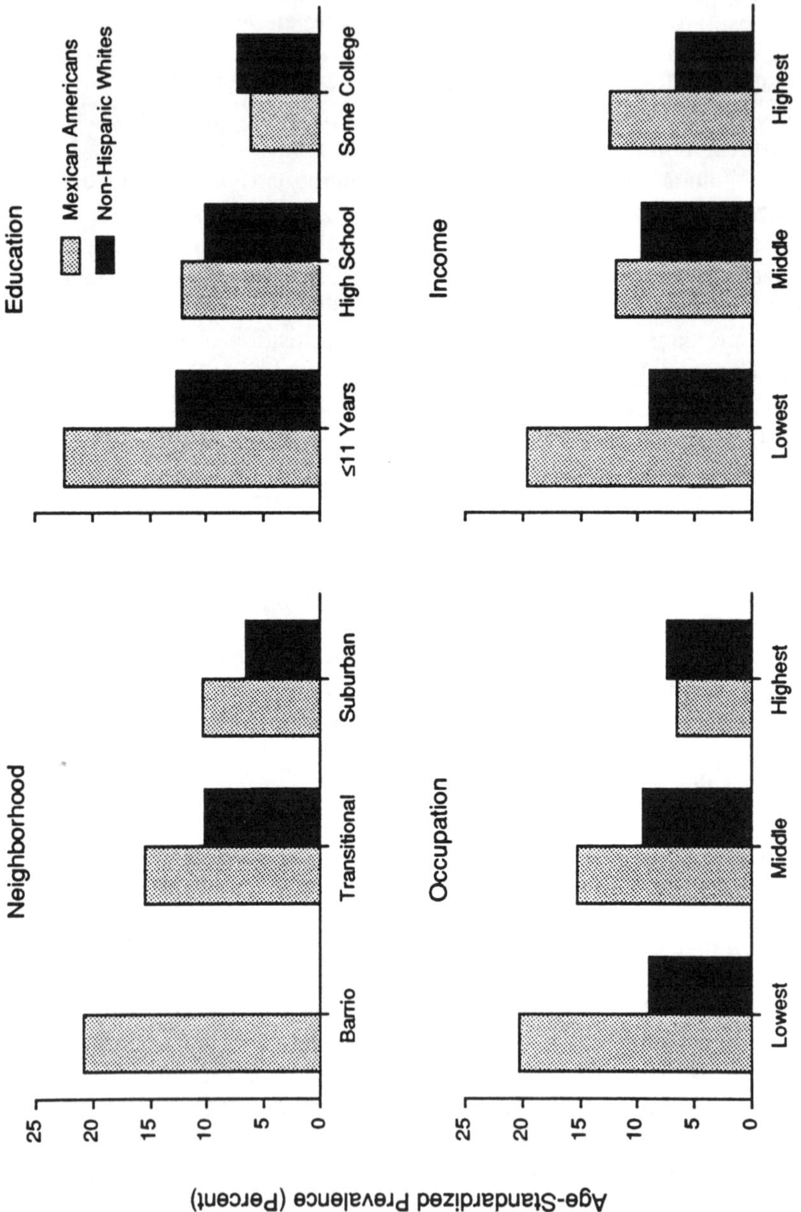

Fig. 1. Prevalence of clinical gallbladder disease in Mexican Americans and non-Hispanic whites, according to four measures of socioeconomic status. (Data from reference [2]).

risk of gallbladder disease in persons with a lifetime cigarette consumption of 20 pack-years or more, although the odds ratios were not statistically significant. Additionally, we confirmed the work of others regarding an inverse relationship of serum HDL-cholesterol to gallbladder disease prevalence, and found an increased risk of disease among persons with hypertriglyceridemia [14]. We examined the relation of dietary intake (assessed by 24-hr recall interviews) to gallbladder disease risk (Fig. 2). Our data suggested a small but statistically non-significant risk with high levels of sucrose intake, and, surprisingly, a higher risk among those with high intake of fiber [9].

Our studies and those of others are identifying a number of 'environmental' risk factors for gallbladder disease, many of which are potentially amenable to medical interventions. It is conceivable that the incidence of gallstones could be affected as a result of such efforts. Already, data from

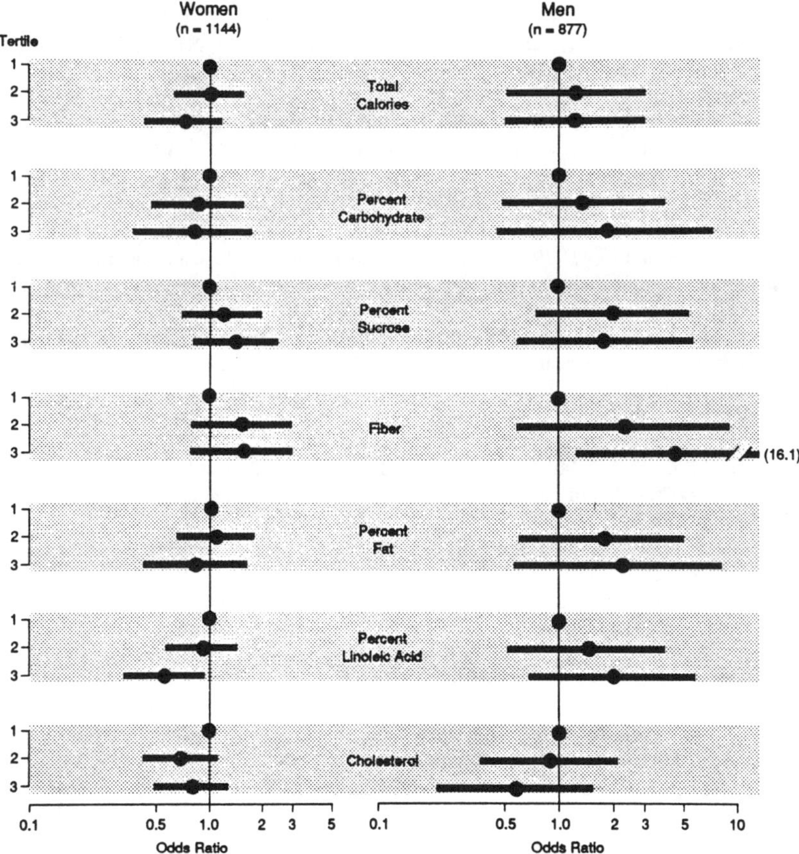

Fig. 2. Odds ratios (with 95% confidence intervals) for clinical gallbladder disease according to tertiles of intake of selected nutrients. For each nutrient, the lowest tertile of intake serves as the reference standard. (Data from reference [9]).

Sweden strongly suggest that gallstone incidence is falling in that country. In the United States, cholecystectomy rates have declined among young and middle aged persons [15]. While the reasons for these changes are uncertain, it is evident that gallstone incidence rates are not immutable. Further investigation of environmental risk factors may suggest measures for the prevention of gallstones.

References

1. Diehl AK, Stern MP, Ostrower VS, Friedman PC (1980): Prevalence of clinical gallbladder disease in Mexican Americans, Anglo, and black women. *South Med J* 73: 438—441, 443.
2. Diehl AK, Rosenthal M, Hazuda HP, Comeaux PJ, Stern MP (1985): Socioeconomic status and the prevalence of clinical gallbladder disease. *J Chron Dis* 38: 1019—1026.
3. Hanis CL, Ferrell RE, Tulloch BR, Schull WJ (1985): Gallbladder disease epidemiology in Mexican Americans in Starr County, Texas. *Am J Epidemiol*, 122: 820—829.
4. Samet JM, Coultas DB, Howard CA, Skipper BJ, Hanis CL (1988): Diabetes, gallbladder disease, obesity, and hypertension among Hispanics in New Mexico. *Am J Epidemiol*, 128: 1302—1311.
5. Arevalo JA, Wollitzer AO, Corporon MB, Larios M, Huante D, Ortiz MT (1987): Ethnic variability in cholelithiasis — an autopsy study. *West J Med* 147: 44—47.
6. Maurer KR, Evérhart JE, Ezzati TM, Johannes RS, Knowler WC, Larson DL, Sanders R, Shawker TH, Roth HP (1989): Prevalence of gallstone disease in Hispanic populations in the United States. *Gastroenterology* 96: 487—492.
7. Diehl AK, Stern MP (1989): Special health problems of Mexican-Americans: obesity, gallbladder disease, diabetes mellitus, and cardiovascular disease. *Adv Intern Med* 34: 73—96.
8. Haffner SM, Diehl AK, Stern MP, Hazuda HP (1989): Central adiposity and gallbladder disease in Mexican Americans. *Am J Epidemiol* 129: 587—595.
9. Diehl AK, Haffner SM, Knapp JA, Hazuda HP, Stern MP (1989): Dietary intake and the prevalence of gallbladder disease in Mexican Americans. *Gastroenterology* 97: 1527—1533.
10. Haffner SM, Diehl AK, Mitchell BD, Stern MP, Hazuda HP (1990): Increased prevalence of clinical gallbladder disease in subjects with non-insulin dependent diabetes mellitus. *Am J Epidemiol* 132: 327—335.
11. Hanis CL, Chakraborty R, Ferrell RE, Schull WJ (1986): Individual admixture estimates: disease associations and individual risk of diabetes and gallbladder disease among Mexican-Americans in Starr County, Texas. *Am J Phys Anthropol* 70: 433—441.
12. Rios-Dalenz J, Takabayashi A, Henson DE, Strom BL, Soloway RD (1983): The epidemiology of cancer of the extra-hepatic biliary tract in Bolivia. *Int J Epidemiol* 12: 156—160.
13. Relethford JH, Stern MP, Gaskill SP, Hazuda HP (1983): Social class, admixture, and skin color variation in Mexican-Americans and Anglo-Americans living in San Antonio, Texas. *Am J Phys Anthropol* 61: 97—102.
14. Diehl AK, Haffner SM, Hazuda HP, Stern MP (1987): Coronary risk factors and clinical gallbladder disease: an approach to the prevention of gallstones? *Am J Public Health* 77: 841—845.
15. Diehl AK (1987): Trends in cholecystectomy rates in the United States. *Lancet* 2: 683.

14. Risk factors for gallstone disease: genetic, ethnic and environmental factors

Z. HALPERN and T. GILAT

Gallstones are a major public health problem in all developed countries. Available evidence suggests that the incidence of gallstones has been rising sharply in recent decades [1, 2]. Like many chronic, non infectious diseases whose incidence increases with age, the pathogenesis of gallstones may be multifactorial. Much has been learned in recent years about factors in bile associated with cholesterol gallstone formation; however the reasons for the rising incidence of gallstones remain unknown. There is evidence to support the existence of all 3 factors which are the subject of the present discussion.

The presence of genetic factors is suggested by the increased familial prevalence of gallstones which has been found in ethnically homogeneous populations living under similar environmental conditions. Surprisingly few studies have been performed on familial factors in gallstone disease and even fewer studies where asymptomatic first degree relatives were investigated. Our study was initiated to assess the prevalence of gallstones in family members of patients with proven gallstones versus a matched control group [3].

A tremendous ethnic variation has been demonstrated in the prevalence of gallstones in studies conducted in various parts of the worlds including in our area, as shown by the considerable differences in the prevalence of gallstones between Jews in Tel Aviv and Arabs in Gaza [4, 5]. In many of these cases it is difficult to disentangle between environmental and ethnic — genetic factors. We chose to study two populations, Jews in Tel Aviv and Arabs in Gaza, who share some genetic traits (like lactase deficiency) as well as geographic and climatic conditions. The main differences were dietary and cultural habits. The purpose of this study was to compare the composition of the diet of these two populations.

Family study

In the early 80's we performed a study of 175 first degree relatives of patients (101 women, 66 men) with proven gallstones versus 200 (87

L. Capocaccia et al. (eds), Recent advances in the epidemiology and prevention of gallstone disease, 95–101.
© 1991 *Kluwer Academic Publishers. Printed in the Netherlands.*

women, 113 men) matched controls. First a patient with gallstones (pro-positus) proven by X-ray, operation or autopsy was identified. Only if he had at least one first degree relative (parents, siblings or children above age 20) was his family included in the study. Almost all were asymptomatic. For each family member examined a control subject were sought and similarly examined. The controls were staff members of the hospital and clinic patients with minor diseases mostly from the dermatologic and ophtalmologic outpatient clinics. We tried to match the control group with the family group by sex, age and community group.

An oral cholecystogram was performed after an overnight fast following the ingestion of 500 mg of iopanoic acid per 20 kg body wt 14 hr before the X-ray examination. In cases of nonvisualization of the gallbladder, the study was repeated using a double dose and if there was again no opacification, an intravenous cholangiogram was performed.

Ultrasound was not widely available at the start of the study.

Results

Gallstones were found in 20.5% of the family group and in 9% of the control group (Fig. 1). The differences were statistically significant for the whole group as well as for women and men separately ($P < 0.01$). Because age, sex, weight and ethnic origin are very important risk factors, the frequency of gallstones in each of these groups was compared separately (Figs. 2—4). The

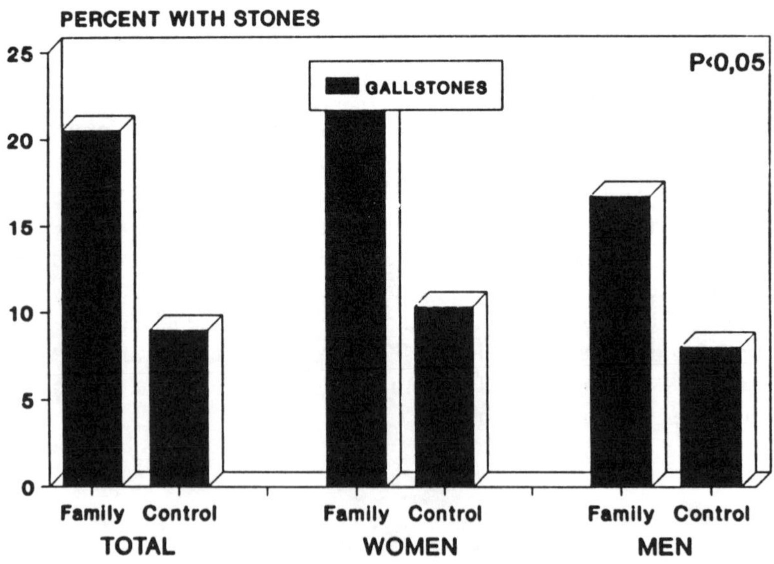

Fig. 1. Frequency of gallstones in family and control groups.

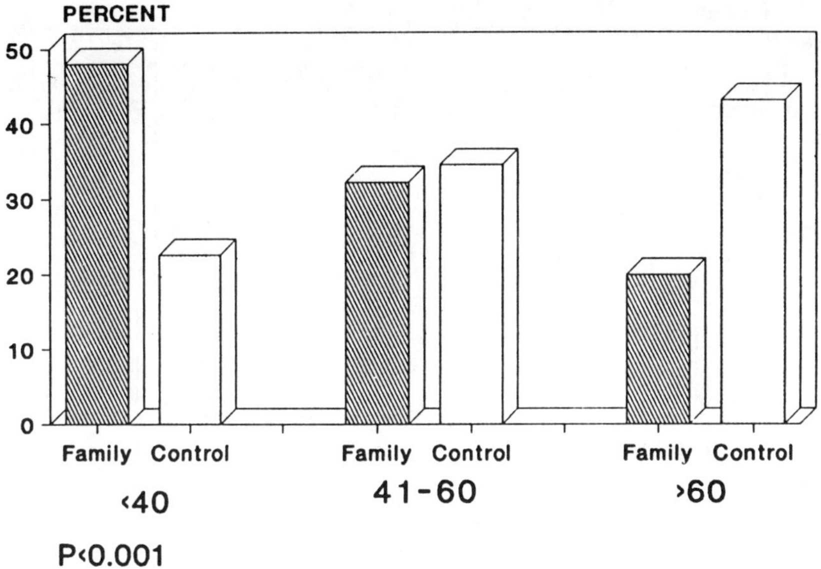

Fig. 2. Age distribution of subjects in family and control groups.

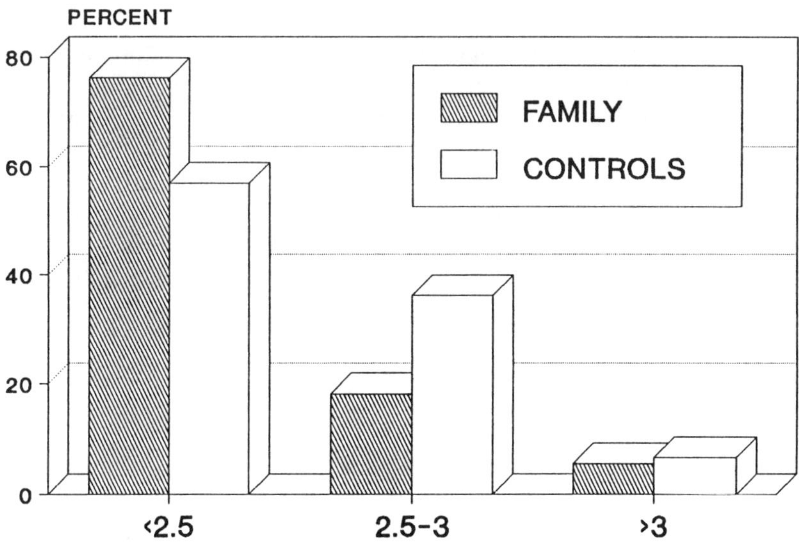

Fig. 3. Relative body weight (Florey) in family and control groups.

difference of gallstone prevalence could not be attributed to a higher load of risk factors in the family group, rather the contrary has emerged. The controls were older and belonged more frequently to the Ashkenazy community group who have a higher prevalence of gallstones.

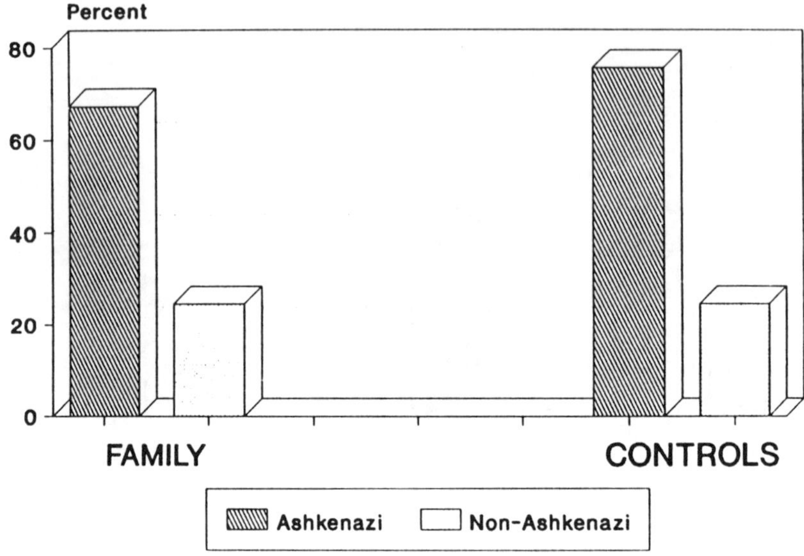

Fig. 4. Community groups distribution in family and control groups.

Discussion

The cause of the increased familial frequency is uncertain. Familial dietary habits could be a factor. However, in view of the negative findings in spouses as found by Van der Linden and others [6, 7], this is very questionable. Gallstones probably take years to develop and are a disease of older age groups. Decades of eating similar food by both husband and wife should show some effect, unless the critical period is in childhood. The epidemiologic evidence of a rising frequency of gallstones disease supports the effect of environmental factors (diet?). These may, however act on genetically susceptible patients.

Dietary study

Previous studies from our department based on autopsy findings have suggested considerable differences in the prevalence of gallstones between Jews in Tel-Aviv and Arabs in Gaza. In the present study we compared the composition of diet in the two populations. X-ray studies of the gallbladder were performed in 424 Arabs from Gaza and 205 Jews from Tel-Aviv. All subjects, above 20 yr of age, were randomly chosen mostly from the outpatients clinic and staff of the hospitals.

Dietary histories were personally elicited from each subject by 24-hr recall. All calculations related to nutrient content of foods were performed by computer using local food composition tables.

Results

Gallstones were significantly more frequent in Jews than in Arabs (Fig. 5). Data were analyzed from both the x-ray and the autopsy study (Fig. 6). Gallstones were significantly more frequent in Jews mainly because of the much higher frequency in the above 60 age group. The daily consumption of

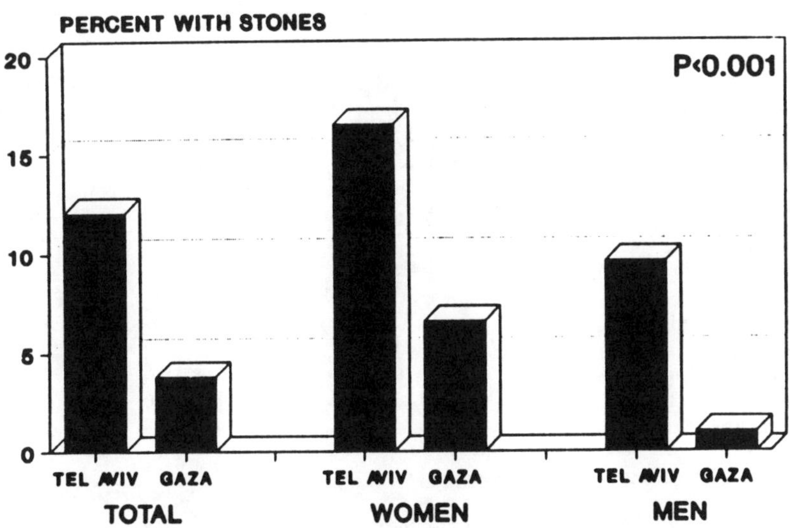

Fig. 5. Frequency of gallstones in Tel-Aviv and Gaza.

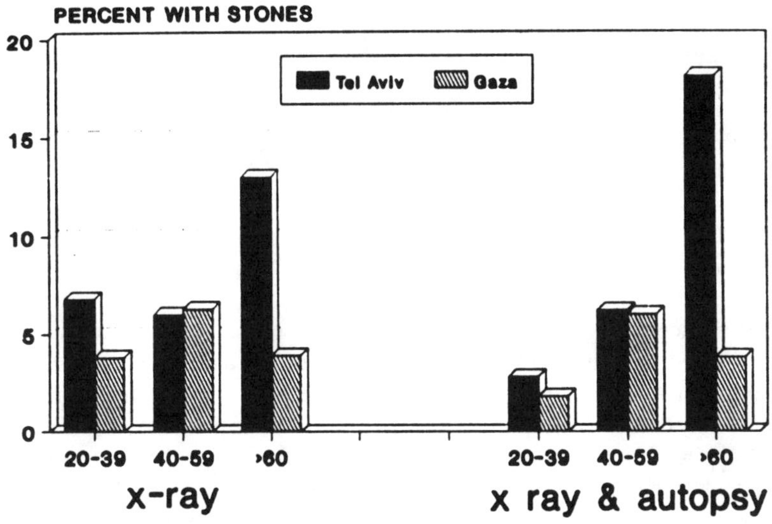

Fig. 6. Percent of subjects with gallstones in Tel-Aviv and Gaza (X-ray and autopsy data).

various food items is shown in Table 1. Energy, Carbohydrate and fiber intake was higher in Gaza. The consumption of unsaturated fats was greater in Gazans and their P/S ratio was higher. There were also differences in vitamin and mineral consumption. Overweight was more frequent among women in Gaza. The average number of living children was 1.8 in Tel-Aviv and 6.2 in Gaza.

Table 1. Daily intake of food constituents (mean ± SEM).

	Tel-Aviv	Gaza	P
Major food constituents			
Energy (calories)	2110.6 ± 57.6	2548.9 ± 68.4	<0.01
Fat (gm)	89.9 ± 3.3	97.8 ± 3.5	NS
Protein (gm)	92.2 ± 2.2	94.6 ± 2.9	NS
Carbohydrate (gm)	230.7 ± 7.8	323.0 ± 10.1	<0.01
Water (gm)	957.3 ± 27.6	975.4 ± 32.1	NS
Fiber (gm)	18.7 ± 0.6	29.3 ± 1.0	<0.01
Fatty acids and cholesterol			
Cholesterol (mg)	411.1 ± 21.8	370.8 ± 25.6	NS
Polyunsaturated (gm)	19.6 ± 10.6	23.6 ± 10.5	<0.01
Monounsaturated (gm)	31.8 ± 13.4	36.7 ± 16.6	<0.05
Saturated (gm)	32.4 ± 14.2	29.4 ± 12.3	NS
P/S	0.7 ± 0.1	0.9 ± 0.1	<0.05
Minerals			
Mg (mg)	207.5 ± 7.0	220.1 ± 10.3	NS
Ca (mg)	659.3 ± 33.8	520.7 ± 26.5	<0.01
Fe (mg)	12.0 ± 0.4	14.8 ± 0.6	<0.01
Zn (mg)	9.3 ± 0.3	9.5 ± 0.3	NS
Vitamins			
Carotene (μg)	2993.8 ± 215	4345.1 ± 212	<0.01
Retinol (μg)	538.5 ± 27.7	207.9 ± 21.7	<0.01
Vit C (mg)	93.8 ± 5.7	108.1 ± 5.2	<0.05
Thiamine (mg)	0.8 ± 0.1	1.1 ± 0.1	<0.01

Discussion

The differences in gallstone prevalence were quite remarkable. However, these differences were entirely due to the older age group. Assuming a correlation between diet and gallstones these data may interpreted in two ways: (1) The diet of Arabs in Gaza leads to a lesser prevalence of gallstones in the older population because it takes years for factors in the diet to produce their effect. (2) It is not the present diet which is important, but rather the diet eaten decades ago by the subjects who are at present over 60 yr old.

There is evidence to suggest that the diet consumed decades ago was much poorer in calories.

Our data illustrate some of the difficulties in correlating diet and gallstones. Many differences in diet composition were found between residents of Tel-Aviv and Gaza. How is one to decide which of these differences has a bearing, if any, on the differences in the prevalence of gallstones. Until more data emerge from future studies, these differences should be noted, however their significance must remain speculative.

Our results demonstrate an increased familial incidence of gallstones which may be due to genetic factors. The second part of the study illustrates the difficulties in attributing proven differences in the prevalence of gallstones to various dietary habits.

Acknowledgements

The authors want to thank to staff members of the Shifa hospital and Rimal Clinic in Gaza and the Ichilov hospital in Tel-Aviv for their help and cooperation.

References

1. Zahor Z, Sternby NH, Kagan A, Uemura K, Vanecek R, Vichert AM (1974): Frequency of cholelithiasis in Prague and Malmo. *Scand J Gastroenterol* 9: 3—7.
2. Kalos A, Delidou A, Kordosis TH, Archimandritis A, Gaganis A, Agnelopoulos B (1977): The incidence of gallstones in Greece: an autopsy study. *Acta Hepato-Gastroenterol* 24: 20—3.
3. Gilat T, Feldman C, Halpern Z, Dan M, Bar-Meir S (1983): An increased familial frequency of gallstones. *Gastroenterology* 84: 242—6.
4. Gilat T, Margoulies JY, Loewenthal M, Meir J, Karplus H (1978): The epidemiology of gallstones in Tel-Aviv area. *G Gastroenterol Endoscop* 1: 105—12.
5. Gilat T, Horwitz C, Halpern Z, Bar Itzhak A, Feldman C (1985): Gallstones and diet in Tel Aviv and Gaza. *Am J Clin Nutr* 41: 336—42.
6. Van der Linden W, Westlin J (1966): The familial occurrence of gallstone disease. II. Occurrence in husbands and wives. *Acta Genet Stat Med* 16: 377—82.
7. Friedman GD, Kannel WB, Dawber TR (1966): The epidemiology of gallbladder disease: observation in the Framingham study. *J Chron Dis* 19: 273—92.

15. Aging and gallstone disease

F. LIRUSSI, G. NASSUATO, D. PASSERA, S. TOSO,
R. M. IEMMOLO and L. OKOLICSANYI

Epidemiology and genetic aspects

In the past, autopsy studies have shown a clear relationship between an increased prevalence of gallstone disease (GD) and increasing age, especially in women [1—3].

Recently, three epidemiologial studies — one from great Britain and two from Italy — have confirmed these data [4—6]. The South Wales study was based on cholecystography and examined a population of about 1000 individuals with an age range of 45 to 69 yr, living in an industrial area. In contrast, the two Italian studies (the GREPCO study in Rome and the Sirmione study) included a larger population (approx. 2000 people each) with a wider age range (18—20 to 64—65 yr) and were therefore comparable between one another. Moreover, both were based on ultrasonography for screening of GD.

The results of the GREPCO and the Sirmione studies showed that age, female sex, obesity and hypertriglyceridemia were associated with an increased prevalene of GD. In particular, in the Sirmione study, GD accounted for 2.1% between 18 and 29 yr, and 19.8% between 50 and 65 yr, the risk of developing gallstones being four times higher in older (40—65 yr) than in younger subjects (18—39 yr) [7].

Preliminary data from the MICOL Study (Multicenter Italian study on Epidemiology of Cholelithiasis) clearly indicate the influence of age and female sex on the prevalence of GD in Italy. The prevalence increases steadily with age and reaches a maximum in the oldest age groups (65—69 yr): 19.3% in men and 31.7% in women.

The MICOL Study examined more than 33000 subjects spread over 18 centers throughout Italy.

Recent data obtained from a cross-sectional study of a suburban Padua population (Montegrotto Terme), consisting of 2978 subjects, are in keeping with the results of the MICOL study. Figure 1 shows the influence of age and sex on the prevalence of gallbladder stones in the subjects examined in the Montegrotto area. As expected, the percentage of individuals with

L. Capocaccia et al. (eds), Recent advances in the epidemiology and prevention of gallstone disease, 103—111.
© 1991 *Kluwer Academic Publishers. Printed in the Netherlands.*

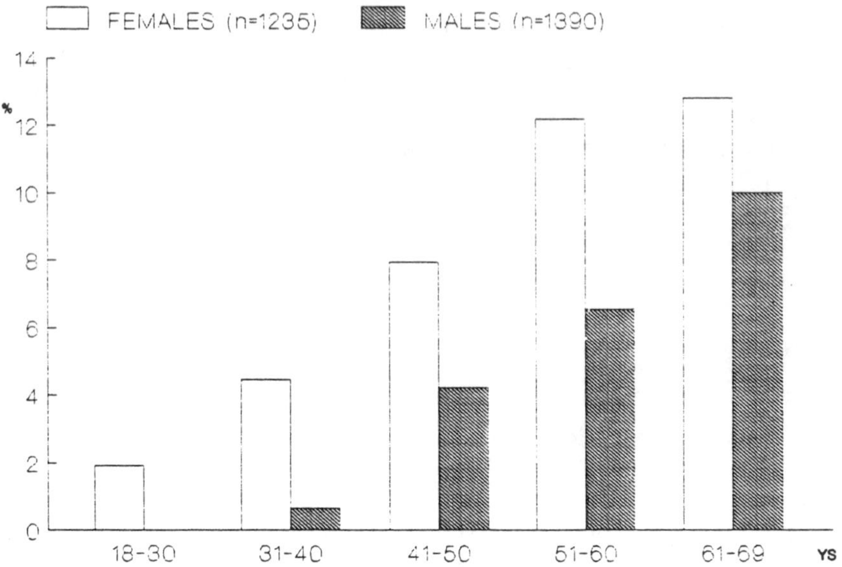

Fig. 1. Prevalence of gallstones in males and females in different age groups in a suburban Padua area (Montegrotto Terme).

gallstones increased progressively with age and reached a maximum of 10% and 12.8% in men and women aged 61—69, respectively.

Cholecystectomy was rare in males less than 40 yr of age and increased up-to a value of about 6% in elderly men (Fig. 2). In contrast, the rate of cholecystectomy tended to level off in women over 40 yr to a value of about 8—9% (Fig. 2). When the prevalence of gallstone disease (gallstones + cholecystectomy) was evaluated in the Montegrotto population, the results in the subjects aged 61—69 were: 15.8 and 21.8% in males and females, respectively.

Although these percentages are somewhat lower than those obtained in the MICOL Study, it must be pointed out that in the Montegrotto survey, the population was divided in 10-yr, and not 5-yr, age-groups.

Thus, the epidemiology studies of the 1980s are largely confirmatory of the autopsy studies, carried out mainly in the 1960s and 1970s, as regards the prevalence of GD in relation to age, at least in the Caucasian population.

Although a relationship between increased prevalence and incidence of GD with increasing age is well documented, genetic factors seem to play an important role only in well-defined ethnic groups such as the Pima Indians of Arizona and the inhabitants of Chile. In the Pima Indians gallstones affect about 75% of adult women and 45% of adult men [8]. Diabetes mellitus, arthritis and some types of eye disease are also very common in this community [8].

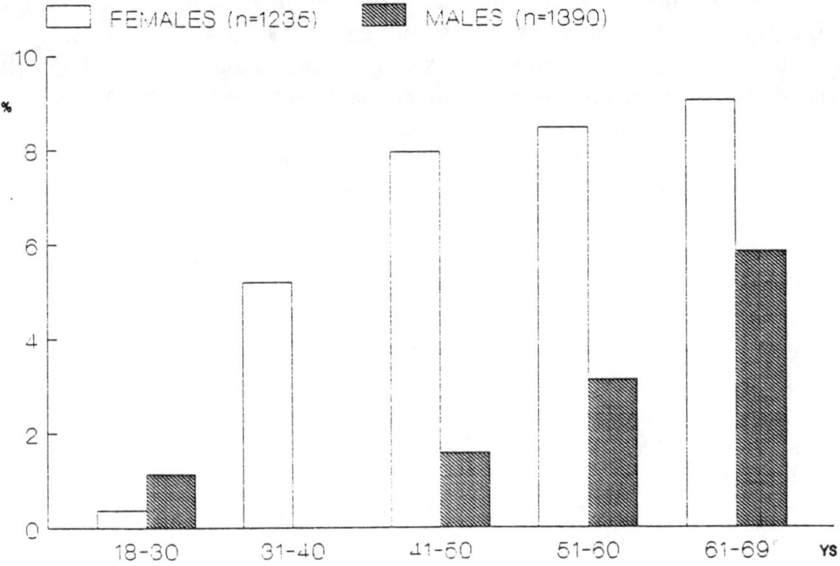

Fig. 2. Prevalence of cholecystectomy in males and females in different age groups in a suburan Padua area (Montegrotto Terme).

In Chileans, a survey carried out on a total of 625 subjects living in a suburban area of Santiago, showed that 17% of the men and 51% of the women over 20 yr of age had gallstones, suggesting an early appearance of GD in this population [9]. These results, however, are difficult to interpret since they are not based on a survey including a general population and do not take into account the prevalence of GD in the oldest age groups.

Aging and biliary lipid metabolism

There is experimental evidence that bile acid metabolism is affected by the aging process. Kitani et al. [10] observed that the transport maximum (T_m) of taurocholate and tauroursodeoxycholate were significantly impaired in old male Wistar rats when compared to those observed in young animals.

Similar results have been reported in the rat with respect to the biliary excretion of chenodeoxycholic and beta-muricholic acids [11]. Moreover, the biliary excretion of bile acids is affected by aging more than the uptake process of these compounds [12], and since bile acids are the major determinants of bile flow, basal bile volume too declines with increasing age [13].

Although the results of animal studies cannot be simply extrapolated to man, the age-related changes of bile acid metabolism, if present in humans, may have no clinical relevance in healthy elderly subjects. In fact, the plasma-to-bile transport systems are very efficient and work normally well below the saturation rates. However, an impaired transport of bile acids through the liver in the aged, might adversely affect the course, and perhaps delay the recovery, of cholestatic jaundice in old patients.

Whether or not these changes may be clinically important, at least two questions arise. Does the entire excretory function of the liver deteriorate with increasing age, likewise the renal function? Alternatively, does the aging process affect specifically the metabolism of one or more of the biliary lipids in the liver?

The findings that in aging rats the biliary T_m of conjugated sulphobromophtalein and ouabain are impaired [13, 14] would support the first hypothesis. However, recent studies of bile acid and cholesterol metabolism in man suggest that hepatic synthesis and the biliary excretion of these compounds are specifically affected by the aging process.

Angelin and co-workers [15] measured cholic acid prodution rate in 38 healthy individuals in relation to age, using Lindstedt's isotope dilution technique and found an inverse relationship between age and bile acid synthesis in both sexes.

In another study, Bertolotti et al. [16] measured the activity of hepatic 7-α-hydroxylase, the rate limiting enzyme for bile acid synthesis, in normal individuals of varying age, and showed a significant inverse correlation between age and 7-α-hydroxylation rates.

It is well-known that bile acids represent the most important conversion product of cholesterol metabolism in the liver. Thus, a reduced availability of cholesterol in the hepatocytes would in turn result in a smaller fraction of cholesterol being converted to bile acids. Experimental data in both animals and man suggest that the postulated decreased intra-hepatic pool of cholesterol is probably due to an age-dependent reduced expression of hepatic LDL receptors for cholesterol of extra-hepatic origin [11, 17].

Finally, if less cholesterol is converted to bile acids with increasing age, more cholesterol should be available for secretion in bile. Indeed, this has been demonstrated by Einarsson and co-workers [17] who found a significant relationship between age and hepatic secretion of cholesterol. These authors calculated that an extra amount of 20—30 μmoles of cholesterol would be available for biliary secretion each hour in a 60-yr old man when compared with a 20-yr old subject (assuming that cholesterol synthesis is unchanged).

Thus, in the elderly, bile acid synthesis is reduced, biliary cholesterol output is increased, whereas both bile acid and phospholipid secretions are not [17]. As a result, the cholesterol saturation of bile increases with increasing age, and that is true in both men and women [17].

Bile acid composition also changes with age. Leiss et al. [18] and Roda et al. [19] reported a significant increase in the percentage of biliary deoxycholate in the elderly. First, since deoxycholic acid is a secondary bile acid which is formed in the intestine by bacterial enzyme dehydroxylation of cholic acid, an excessive growth of intestinal flora would occur even in apparently healthy elderly subjects. Indirect evidence of bacterial overgrowth in the aged gut has been provided by Hellemans and co-workers [20] using the 14-C-glycocholic acid breath test. These authors found an abnormally high cumulative percentage of $14\text{-}CO_2$ in the expired air of both healthy and ill elderly subjects, which, however, tended to decrease after antibiotic therapy.

Secondly, the increased fraction of the highly detergent deoxycholate in bile could be responsible, at least in part, for the enhanced concentration of biliary cholesterol observed in the elderly [17].

In summary, the results of the above reported studies of bile lipid metabolism, all agree that bile becomes saturated in cholesterol with increasing age. This phenomenon represents a prerequisite for the nucleation of cholesterol crystals. However, other factors including the presence of nucleating agents, the absence of antinucleating substances, changes of biliary pH and viscosity, an unbalance between vesicle and micellar carriers of cholesterol in bile, and gallbladder hypomotility, all seem important for cholesterol gallstone formation [21].

Khalil and co-workers [22] investigated the effect of aging on gallbladder contraction and cholecystokinin (CCK) release. They studied 29 gallstone-free volunteers who were divided into two age groups: 14 young subjects between 22 and 42 yr of age and 15 older subjects aged 60—84 yr. The gallbladder volume was measured by means of ecotomography before and after oral corn oil administration, and CCK concentrations were determined by radioimmunoassay. The authors found that the sensitivity of the gallbladder to CCK diminished with age but this effect was counterbalanced by an increased release of CCK, so that gallbladder emptying differed little in the aged.

This study further emphasizes the role of altered bile acid and bile lipid compostion of bile in promoting the formation of biliary stones in the elderly, in the absence of age-related alterations of gallbladder emptying.

Characteristics of gallstones in the aged

Van Erpecum and co-workers [23] in the Netherlands examined the composition of gallbladder stones in relation to age in 116 patients referred to their department for elective cholecystectomy. They showed that 40% of gallstone patients over 50 yr of age had pigment stones, whereas all the patients younger than 50 yr had cholesterol stones, and suggested that the relative frequency of pigment and cholesterol stones varies with increasing age.

With the aim of gaining information on the characteristics of biliary stones and the gallbladder in relation to age, we studied a total of 125 patients with silent stones and divided them into two groups according to age under or over 60 yr (Table 1). We found that 46% of the patients over 60 yr had stones with a diameter larger than 15 mm, a generally accepted cut-off point for bile acid therapy, whereas only approximately 20% of the younger subjects had large stones. Interestingly, there were no singificant differences between the two age groups in the percentage of patients who were overweight, and of those with calcific rimmed stones, or with abnormal gallbladder function (as assessed by oral cholecystography) [24]. Thus, gallstone size tends to increase with age, whereas neither the biliary secretion of calcium nor the capacity of the gallbladder wall to concentrate the contrast medium seem to be affected by the aging process.

Table 1. Characteristics of gallstones and gallbladder function in 125 patients with silent stones under or over 60 yr of age. IBW = ideal body weight.

Age groups	Stone diam. > 15 mm	No gallbladder opacification	Calcific RIM	BW > 130% IBW
< 60 yr	20.4%	20.8%	9.3%	6.6%
> 60 yr	46.4%	16.2%	8.3%	6.4%
p	< 0.05	n.s.	n.s.	n.s.

Recently, Mok and co-workers [25], measuring the profiles of 14-C incorporated in gallbladder, and common bile duct, stones showed that grow rates of stones varied between 1 and 4 mm yr^{-1} both in symptomatic and asymptomatic patients.

A final point of discussion regards the possibility of gallstone dissolution by oral bile acid therapy in the elderly.

As a background study [26], we first treated 135 symptomatic gallstone patients of varying age with ursodeoxycholic acid (8-10 mg/kg/day) or chenodeoxycholic acid (13—15 mg/kg/day) for 6—24 months and evaluated the influence of different variables, including age, on gallstone dissolution by means of the univariate and the multivariate analyses. The univariate analysis indicated that age less than 40 yr was a significant factor which favoured complete gallstone dissolution. However, when the more powerful multivariate regression analysis was applied, factors other than age appeared to influence significantly the outcome of bile acid treatment.

These results emphasize that age has to be considered together with other variables and not as a single risk factor, and also that advanced age, per se, is not a negative 'prognostic' factor in terms of gallstone dissolution.

On the basis of the previous results, we treated 26 elderly gallstone patients with either ursodeoxycholic acid or chenodeoxycholic acid at the same dosage as reported above, and compared the outcome of gallstone dissolution with a younger gallstone population. When ursodeoxycholic acid was given, the response rate, with respect to partial + complete dissolution, was similar in the two age groups (about 55%), whereas it was significantly lower in the elderly patients treated with chenodeoxycholic acid (27% versus 47%) [27]. Thus, ursodeoxycholic acid or perhaps a combination of 'urso + cheno' seem preferable to chenodeoxycholic alone in symptomatic elderly patients with GD.

Conclusions

The results of the reviewed studies and our own data can be summarized as following: (i) the prevalence of gallstone disease increases with age and is higher in females than in males in the Caucasian population; (ii) possible pathogenetic mechanisms include increased cholesterol secretion and reduced bile acid synthesis related to age; (iii) the characteristics of gallstones in the elderly are compatible with a long-standing disease; (iv) advanced age does not represent a contraindication to oral bile acid therapy, although other types of non-surgical approaches, for example shock-wave lithotripsy, may also be indicated in elderly gallstone patients, due to the tendency of the stones to grow in size with increasing age.

Acknowledgements

Thanks are due to Mrs Anna Zanninovich who kindly typed the manuscript.

References

1. Stitnimankarn T (1960): The necropsy incidence of gallstones in Thailand. *Am J Med Sci* 243: 349—352.
2. Zahor Z, Sternhy NH, Kagan A, Nemura K, Vanecek R, Vichert AM (1974): Frequency of cholelithiasis in Prague and Malmoe. An autopsy study, *Scand J Gastroent* 9: 3—7.
3. Lindstrom CG (1977): Frequency of gallstone disease in a well-defined Swedish population. *Scand J Gastroent* 12: 341—346.
4. Bainton D, Davies GT, Evans KT, Gravelle IH (1976): Gallbladder disease. Prevalence in a South Wales industrial town. *N Engl J Med* 294: 1147—1149.
5. Attili AF and the Rome Group for the Epidemiology and Prevention of Cholelithiasis (GREPCO) (1987): *Am J Dig Dis* 32: 349—353.
6. Barbara L, Sama C, Morselli Labate AM et al. (1987): A population study on the prevalence of gallstone disease: the Sirmione Study. *Hepatology* 7: 913—917.
7. Sama C, Frabboni R, Barbara L, Festi D et al. (1988): Associated and risk factors of gallstones disease: The 'Sirmione Study'. Presented at the *International Meeting on 'Pathochemistry, Pathophysiology and Pathomechanics of the Biliary System*, p. 139, March 14—16, Bologna.
8. Knowler WC, Carraher MJ, Pettitt DJ, Bennett PH (1984): Epidemiology of cholelithiasis in the Pima Indians, pp. 15—22 in: Capocaccia L, Ricci G, Angelico F, Angelico M,

Attili, AF (eds), *Epidemiology and Prevention of Gallstone Disease*, Lancaster, MTP Press.

9. Covarrubias C, Valdivieso V, Nervi F (1984): Epidemiology of gallstone disease in Chile, pp. 26—30 in: Capocaccia L, Ricci G, Angelico F, Angelico M, Attili AF (eds), *Epidemiology and Prevention of Gallstone Disease*, Lancaster, MTP Press.

10. Kitani K, Kanai S, Ohta M, Sato Y (1986): Differing transport maxima values for taurine conjugated bile salts in rats and hamsters. *Am J Physiol* 251: G852—G858.

11. Uchida K, Matsubara T, Ishikawa Y, Ito N (1982): Age-related changes in cholesterol-bile acid metabolism and hepatic mixed function oxidase activities in rats, pp. 192—211 in: Kitani K (ed), *Liver and Aging — 1982. Liver and Drugs*, Amsterdam, Elsevier/North-Holland, Biomedical Press.

12. Kroker R, Hegner D, Anwer MS (1980): Altered hepatobiliary transport of taurocholic acid in aged rats. *Mech Age Dev* 12: 367—373.

13. Kanai S, Kitani K, Fujita 5, Kitagawa H (1985): The hepatic handling of sulfobromoph-thalein in aging Fisher-344 rats: in vivo and in vitro studies. *Arch Gerontol Geriatr* 4: 73—85.

14. Ohta M, Kanai S, Sato Y, Kitani K (1988): Age-dependent decrease in the hepatic uptake and biliary excretion of ouabain in rats. *Biochem Pharmacol* 37: 935—942.

15. Angelin B, Berglund L, Einarsson K, Ericsson S, Eriksson M (1987): Disturbances of bile acid metabolism and abnormalities of lipoprotein turnover, pp. 277—280 in: Paumgartner G, Stiehl A and Gerok W (eds), *Bile Acids and the Liver*, Lancaster, MTP Press.

16. Bertolotti M, Bertolotti S, Menozzi D, Iori E, Carulli N (1989): Ageing and bile acid metabolism: studies on 7-α-hydroxylation of cholesterol in humans, pp. 75—78 in: Paumgartner G, Gerok W (eds), *Trends in Bile Acid Research*, Lancaster, Kluwer Academic Publishers.

17. Einarsson K, Nilsell K, Leijd B, Angelin B (1985): Influence of age on secretion of cholesterol and synthesis of bile acids by the liver. *N Engl J Med*, 313: 277—282.

18. Leiss O, Becker M, von Bergman K (1987): Effect of age and individual endogenous bile acids on biliary lipid secretions in humans, pp. 217—224 in: Paumgartner G, Stiehl A, Gerok V (eds), *Bile Acids and the Liver*, Lancaster, MTP Press.

19. Roda E, Bazzoli F, Mazzella G, Villanova L et al. (1987): Effect of age and sex on bile acid metabolism and biliary lipid secretion in normal subjects and gallstone patients, pp. 225—227 in: Paumgartner G, Stiehl A, Gerok W (eds), *Bile Acids and the Liver*, Lancaster, MTP Press.

20. Hellemans J, Joosten E, Ghoos Y, Carchon H, Vantrappen G, Pelemans W, Rutgeerts P (1984). Positive $^{14}CO_2$ bile acid breath test in elderly people. *Age Ageing* 13: 138—143.

21. Carey MC (1989): Formation of cholesterol gallstones: the new paradigms, pp. 259—282 in: Paumgartner G, Gerok W (eds), *Trends in Bile Acid Research*, Lancaster, Kluwer Academic Publishers.

22. Khalil T, Walker JP, Wiener I et al. (1985): Effect of aging on gallbladder contraction and release of cholecystokinin-33 in humans. *Surgery*, 98: 423—429.

23. Van Erpecum, KJ, Van Berge Henegouwen GP, Stoelwinder B, Stolk MF, Eggink WF, Govaert WHA (1988): Cholesterol and pigment gallstone disease in the Netherlands: epidemiological data and comparison of the reliability of bile tests for the differentiation between both stone types. Presented at the *International Meeting on 'Pathochemistry, Pathophysiology and Pathomechanics of the biliary system*, p. 153, March 14—16, Bologna.

24. Lirussi F, Orlando R, Iemmolo RM, Nassuato G, Okolicsanyi L (1989): Asymptomatic gallstone disease: how many patients are eligible for bile acid therapy? Presented at *Ist International Symposium on Biliary Physiology and Diseases*, Strategies for the Treatment of Hepatobiliary Diseases, Lugano, June 15—17, p. 44.

25. Mok HYI, Druffel ERM, Rampone WM (1986): Chronology of cholelithiasis. *N Engl J Med* 17: 1075—1077.

26. Lirussi F, Iemmolo RM, Piccoli A, Orlando R, Nassuato G, Strazzabosco M, Muraca M, Okolicsanyi L (1988): Evaluation of prognostic factors of medical dissolution of cholesterol gallstones using Cox's multivariate regression model. *Curr Ther Res* 43: 128—142.
27. Lirussi F, Iemmolo RM, Orlando R, Nassuato G, Strazzabosco M, Okolicsanyi L (1987): Bile acid treatment of cholesterol cholelithiasis in the elderly. Presented at *Symposium on Aging in Liver and Gastro-Intestinal Tract*, p. 37, 10—12 June, Titisee.

16. Gallstone prevalence in obese women: pathogenic role of hyperlipoproteinaemia and gallbladder motility

M. ACALOVSCHI, A. GEORECEANU, R. BADEA, and D. BLENDEA

Summary

Gallstone (GS) prevalence in 115 obese women and 132 controls matched for age was established by ultrasonography. Gallstones were detected in 41.7% of the obese and in 16.6% of the non-obese women ($p < 0.01$). Among the severely obese (over 150% ideal weight), 47.6% had GS, as compared to 40.3% of the moderately obese ($p > 0.90$). The age of onset of obesity was before 20 years (early onset obesity) in 44.8% of the obese with GS and in 21.1% of the obese women without GS ($p < 0.02$). This finding suggests that age of onset of obesity may affect the prevalence of GS in the obese women.

Hyperlipoproteinaemia (HLP) was present in 25% non-obese and in 40.6% obese women ($p < 0.05$). Type IV HLP was significantly more frequent in the obese (34.2%) than in the non-obese (15%) ($p < 0.05$). In the female patients with GS, we found a higher prevalence of HLP in the obese (54%) versus the non-obese (26.3%) ($p < 0.05$). In spite of these findings, there were no differences concerning HLP prevalence in the obese with and those without GS, indicating obesity as the major risk factor for GS in these patients.

The present investigation was also undertaken to obtain further information on GB motility in obese women. We found a GB fasting volume significantly larger in obese women (40.2 ± 16.3 cc) versus controls (27.8 ± 9.0 cc) ($p < 0.01$). As it positively correlated with relative body weight, the larger GB volume could be simply due to the increased body size. The similar GB ejection fraction in the obese ($60.1 \pm 14.6\%$) and controls ($58.9 \pm 19.2\%$) without GS suggests that GB hypocontractility does not represent a lithogenic risk factor in obesity.

Among the metabolic disorders with lithogenic risk, obesity and hyperlipoproteinaemia (HLP) are the most important. Obese patients have a higher relative concentration of biliary cholesterol and an increased saturation of gallbladder (GB) bile with cholesterol as compared to healthy controls matched for sex, age and serum lipids [1, 2]. Non-obese persons

L. Capocaccia et al. (eds), Recent advances in the epidemiology and prevention of gallstone disease, 113–120.
© 1991 Kluwer Academic Publishers. Printed in the Netherlands.

with primary HLP (type IIb and IV) were also reported to have a super-saturated bile and an increased prevalence of gallstones (GS) [3]. Parity and use of oral contraceptives represent additional lithogenic risk factors in women [4, 5]. Consecutively, biliary disease is the third most frequent obesity-related illness in women [6].

The pathogenic role of GB motility and biliary stasis in GS formation has assumed increasing importance in recent years. Theoretically, GB stasis may allow supersaturated bile to nucleate, crystalize and form stones.

The aim of the present study was to appreciate GS prevalence in obese women and to correlate it with the relative body weight, the age of onset of obesity and with the associated HLP. The investigation was also undertaken to obtain further information on GB motility in obese versus non-obese women.

Material and methods

The study was carried out in 115 obese women (relative body weight over 120% ideal weight) and in 132 non-obese women (controls) matched for age. All gave written informed consent to the study. Ultrasonography of the GB was performed in all patients using a Bruël and Kjaer type 3501 scanner with a 3.5 MHz transducer. The prevalence of GS was calculated in obese and non-obese persons, for each age-group. Statistical analysis was performed using the Chi-square test with Yates correction.

In order to evaluate whether the age of onset of obesity might affect the prevalence of gallstones in obese women, these were divided into two groups: with early onset obesity (onset before 20 yr of age) and with maturity onset obesity (onset after 20 yr).

Blood specimens from fasting subjects (70 obese and 40 non-obese women) were prelevated for measurement of concentrations of total serum cholesterol, triglycerides and lipoproteins. The prevalence of normolipemia and HLP was comparatively calculated in both groups.

Gallbladder fasting volume (FV) was sonographically measured in 21 obese and 14 non-obese women using the unique cylinder formula [7]. The percent residual volume (RV) was determined 30 minutes after a standard-ized fatty meal, consisting of two egg-yolks (RV/FV $\times$ 100 = GB ejection fraction). Data were expressed as mean $\pm$ SD. The relationship between fasting GB volume and relative body weight and age was determined by means of the correlation coefficient and the linear regression analysis.

Results

Gallstones were detected in 48 of 115 obese women (41.7%), significantly more frequently than in non-obese women (22 of 132, 16.6%) (p $<$ 0.01).

The prevalence of gallstones progressively increased with age in both groups. It was higher in the obese for all age-groups, but significantly only for younger ages (Table 1).

Among the severely obese women (over 150% ideal weight), 47.6% had GS, comparatively with 40.3% of the moderately obese ($p > 0.90$).

The age of onset of obesity was before 20 years (early onset obesity) in 13 of 29 obese with GS (44.8%) and in 7 of 33 alithiasic obese women (21.2%) ($p < 0.02$).

Hyperlipoproteinaemia was present in 25% non-obese and in 48.6% obese women ($p < 0.05$) (Table 2). Type IV HLP was significantly more frequent in the obese (34.2%) than in the non-obese (15.0%) ($p < 0.05$). We found no statistically significant difference concerning HLP prevalence in the obese with and without GS (Table 3). When analyzing all women with GS, there was a significantly higher prevalence of HLP in the obese (54%) versus non-obese (26.3%) ($p < 0.05$), although HLP IV prevalence did not differ in these two groups (Table 4).

Table 1. Prevalence or gallstones (GS) in obese women and controls.

| Age | Obese women | | | Non-obese women | | | Chi-square |
| (years) | Total | With GS | | Total | With GS | | analysis |
	no	no	%	no	no	%	
20—29	8	3	37.5	7	1	14.2	NS
30—39	11	3	27.2	19	2	10.5	NS
40—49	28	10	35.6	23	2	8.0	$p < 0.05$
50—59	42	20	47.6	36	5	13.6	$p < 0.02$
60—69	18	9	50.0	35	9	25.7	NS
70—79	8	3	37.5	7	2	28.5	NS
80—89	—			3	1	33.3	—
Total	115	48	41.7	132	22	16.6	$p < 0.01$

Table 2. Prevalence of HLP in obese (no = 70) and non-obese (no = 40) women.

| Serum lipids' | Obese women | | Non-obese women | | Chi-square |
profile	no	%	no	%	analysis
Normolipemia	36	51.4	30	75.0	$p < 0.05$
HLP IIa	4	5.7	2	5.0	NS
HLP IIb	4	5.7	2	5.0	NS
HLP IV	24	34.2	6	15.0	$p < 0.05$
HLP V	2	2.9	—		—

Table 3. Prevalence of HLP in the obese women with gallstones (GS) (no = 37) and without GS (no = 33).

Serum lipids' profile	Obese women with GS		Obese women without GS		Chi-square analysis
	no	%	no	%	
Normolipemia	17	45.4	19	57.5	NS
HLP IIa	1	2.7	3	9.0	NS
HLP IIb	3	8.1	1	3.0	NS
HLP IV	15	40.5	9	27.2	NS
HLP V	1	2.7	1	3.0	NS

Table 4. Prevalence of HLP in the lithiasic obese (no = 37) and non-obese (no = 19) women.

Type of HLP	Obese with GS		Non-obese with GS		Chi-square analysis
	no	%	no	%	
IIa	1	2.7	1	5.2	
IIb	3	8.1	—		
IV	15	40.5	4	21.1	
V	1	2.7	—		
Total	20	54.0	5	26.3	p < 0.05

Gallbladder fasting volume was significantly higher in the obese women (40.2 ± 16.3 cc) than in the non-obese (27.8 ± 9.0 cc) ($p < 0.01$) (Fig. 1). It did not correlate with age, but significantly correlated with relative body weight ($r = +0.56$; $p < 0.05$) (Fig. 2). Gallbladder ejection fraction was similar in the obese ($60.1 \pm 14.6\%$) and non-obese women ($58.9 \pm 19.2\%$) without GS.

Discussions

The incidence of biliary disease in obese persons is three to four times greater than that reported in the general population [4, 8—13]. The increased concentration of cholesterol in the bile, making it supersaturated or lithogenic, is the main mechanism which favours the formation of cholesterol stones in obesity [12, 14, 15]. In a previous study, we also found a direct correlation between biliary cholesterol concentration and relative body weight [16]. One recent report [17] suggested that a low concentration of bile acids (and phospholipids) is the major biliary metabolic defect in obesity.

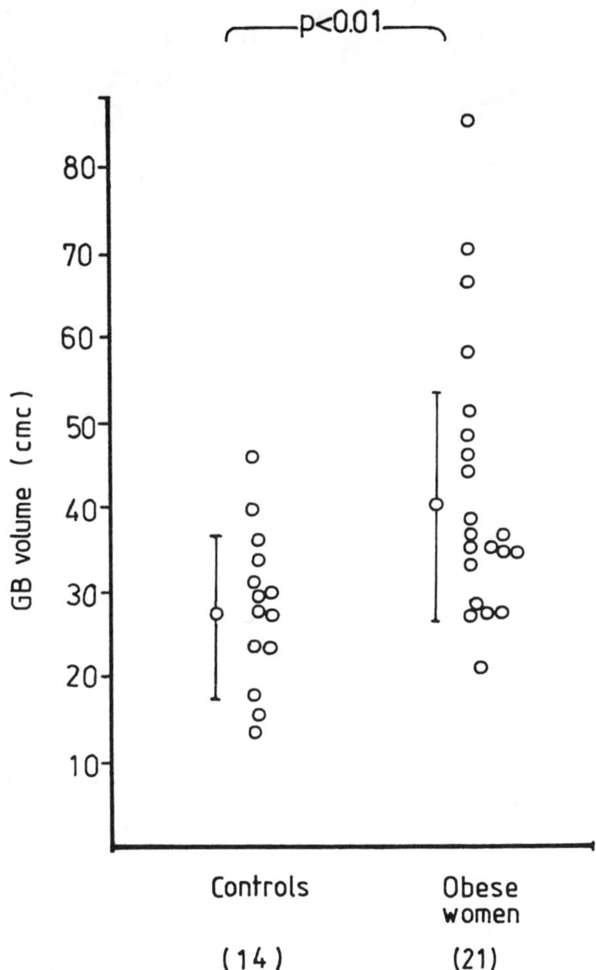

Fig. 1. Gallbladder fasting volume in obese women and controls.

Hyperlipoproteinaemia, especially type IV and IIb, is by now a well-docu-
mented lithogenic factor. The increased prevalence of cholesterol GS in HLP
IV is due to enhanced (even doubled) activity of HMGCOA reductase in the
liver of these patients. Obesity and impaired glucose tolerance are encountered in about 50% of the patients with type IIb and IV HLP, and less
frequently in other types. In a previous investigation, we confirmed that HLP
IV is the most frequent type of HLP in patients with cholesterol GS,
irrespective of their relative body weight, and we found no significant
differences in serum lipids' concentration between GS patients and controls,
except for the triglyceride level [16, 18]. Our data differed from those
mentioning an atherogenic profile of serum lipids in gallstone disease [19]
and were similar to those obtained in female patients by Alvaro et al. [20].

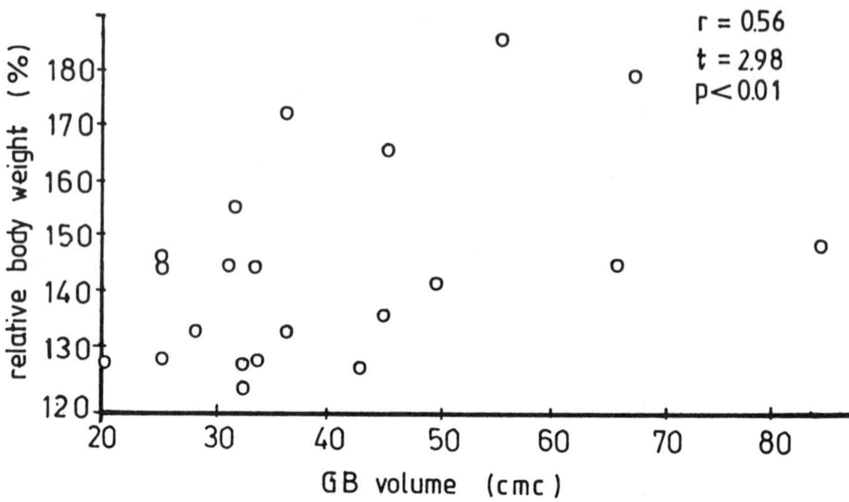

Fig. 2. Correlation of gallbladder fasting volume with relative body weight.

In the present study, we found a significantly higher prevalence of GS in the obese (41.7%) than in the non-obese women (16.6%) (p < 0.01). It progressively increased with age and was higher in the obese women for every decade, but significantly for younger ages, a finding in agreement with other studies [5, 10, 21—23]. In morbidly obese persons, the prevalence is supposed to be more than 40% given the lower sensitivity for GS detection of sonography performed through a large adipose mass [10]. In our study, the prevalence of GS was 40.3% in the moderately obese and 47.6% in the severely obese, a difference without statistical significance.

An original finding of this study was the positive correlation between the age of onset of obesity and the presence of GS (p < 0.02). Age of onset of obesity may, at least in part, affect the prevalence of GS in severe obesity.

As expected, we found a significantly higher prevalence of HLP, especially of HLP IV, in the obese women than in controls. Hyperlipoproteinaemia was also more frequent in the obese with GS than in the controls with GS. In the obese, the prevalence and types of HLP did not differ whether they had or had not GS, indicating obesity as the major risk factor for GS.

The pathogenic role of GB stasis for the development of stones was analyzed in recent years also in the obese [24, 25]. Like these authors, we found a GB fasting volume significantly larger in obese women versus controls. It did not correlate with age, but significantly correlated with relative body weight, a fact observed by Kucio [25] and contested by Marzio [24]. We found a similar GB ejection fraction in the obese and controls without GS, indicating a normal release of CCK or a normal response to CCK at the receptor site in the obese women. Shreiner et al [26] reported a similar GB motility in the obese with and without GS, arguing against an eventual role of GB stasis in GS development in obesity. On the contrary, Marzio et al. [24] observed a significantly blunted GB contractility in obese vs. controls both after the ordinary and low-calorie meal. Data concerning GB motility in obese persons are therefore few and controversed. Our study suggests that GB hypocontractility does not represent a lithogenic risk factor in obesity. The larger GB volume found in our obese women could be simply due to the increased body size, as it positively correlated with relative body weight.

References

1. Bennion LJ, Grundy SM (1978): Risk factors for the development of cholelithiasis. *New Engl J Med* 289: 1161—8.
2. Angelin B, Einarsson K, Everth S, Leijd B (1981): Biliary lipid composition in obesity. *Scand J Gastroenterol* 16: 1015—9.
3. Ahlberg J, Angelin B, Einarsson K, Hellström K, Leijd B (1980): Biliary lipid composition in normo- and hyperlipoproteinaemia. *Gastroenterology* 79: 90—4.
4. Honoré LH (1980): Cholesterol cholelithiasis in adolescent females. Its connection with obesity, parity and oral contraceptive use. A retrospective study of 31 cases. *Arch Surg* 115: 62—4.
5. Lee SS, Wasiljew BK, Lee MJ (1987): Gallstones in women younger than thirty. *J Clin Gastroenterol* 9: 65—9.
6. Rimm AA, Werner LH, Yserloo BV, Bernstein RA (1975): Relationship of obesity and disease in 73 532 weight-conscious women. *Public Health Rep* 90: 44—54.
7. Everson GT, Braverman DZ, Johnson ML, Kern F Jr (1980): A critical evaluation of real-time ultrasonography for the study of gallbladder volume and contraction. *Gastroenterology* 79: 40—6.
8. Friedman GD, Kannel WB, Dawber TR (1966): The epidemiology of gallbladder disease: Observations in the Framingham study. *J Chronic Dis* 19: 273—9.
9. Angel A (1978): Pathophysiologic changes in obesity. *Canad Med Ass J* 119: 1401—11.
10. Amaral JF, Thompson WH (1985): Gallbladder disease in the morbidly obese. *Amer J Surg* 149: 351—7.
11. Mellström D, Asztely M, Svancik J (1988): Gallstones and previous cholecystectomy in 75 year old women in an urban population in Sweden. *Pathochemistry, Pathophysiology and Pathomechanics of the Biliary System. New Strategies for the Treatment of Biliary Tract Disease.* March 14—16, Bologna.
12. Williams CN, Johnston JL (1980): Prevalence of gallstones and risk factors in Caucasian women in a rural Canadian community. *Can Med Ass J* 122: 664—8.
13. Barbara L, Sama C, Taroni F, Rusticali AG, Festi D, Sapio C, Roda E, Banterle C, Puci A, Formentini F, Colasanti S, Nardin F (1987): A population study on the prevalence of gallstone disease: the Sirmione study. *Hepátology* 7: 913—7.
14. Williams CN, Johnston JL, McCarthy S, Field CA (1981): Biliary lipid, bile acid composition and dietary correlations in Micmac Indian women. A population study. *Dig Dis Sci* 26: 42—9.
15. StGeorge CM, Russell JC, Shaffer EA (1989): The influence of obesity on bile secretion and lipid composition in the La/N-corpulent rat. *Gastroenterology* 96: part 2 abstr.
16. Acalovschi M, Suciu A, Florea M, Dumitrascu D, Grigorescu M (1984): Lipides biliaires majeurs et lipides plasmatiques. Etude dans la lithiase biliaire à cholesterol. *Acta Gastroenterol Belg* 67: 381—6.

17. Jazrawi RP, Galatola G, Lanzini A (1988): Gallbladder lipid mass in cholesterol gallstone patients: effect of sex and obesity. *Pathochemistry, Pathophysiology and Pathomechanics of the Biliary System. New Strategies for the Treatment of Biliary Tract Disease.* March 14—16, Bologna.
18. Dumitraşcu D, Acalovschi M, Grigorescu M (1989): *Litiaza biliară.* Bucureşti, Ed. Acad. RSR.
19. Petitti DB, Friedman GD, Klatsky AL (1981): Association of a history of gallbladder disease with a reduced concentration of high-density lipoprotein cholesterol. *New Engl J Med* 304: 1396—8.
20. Alvaro D, Angelico F, Attili AF, Antonini R, Mazzarella B, Corradini SG, Gentile S, Bracci F, Angelico M (1986): Plasma lipid lipoproteins and biliary lipid composition in female gallstone patients. *Biomed Biochim Acta* 45: 761—8.
21. Tucker LE, Tangedahl TN, Newmark S (1982): Prevalence of gallstones in obese Caucasian American women. *Int J Obes* 6: 247—51.
22. Thiet MD, Mittelstaedt CA, Herbit CA, Buckwalter JA (1984): Cholelithiasis in morbid obesity. *South Med J* 77: 415—7.
23. Scragg RKR, McMichael AJ, Baghurst PA (1984): Diet, alcohol, and relative body weight in gallstone disease: a case-control study. *Brit Med J* 288: 1113—9.
24. Marzio L, Capone F, Neri M, Mezzetti A, de Angelis C, Cuccurullo F (1988): Gallbladder kinetics in obese patients. Effect of a regular meal and low-calorie meal. *Dig Dis Sci* 33: 4—9.
25. Kucio C, Besser P, Jonderko K (1988): Gallbladder motor function in obese versus lean females. *Europ J Clin Nutr* 42: 121—4.
26. Shreiner DP, Sarva RP, VanThiel D, Yingvorapant N (1986): Gallbladder function in diabetic patients. *J Nucl Med* 27: 357—60.

17. Serum lipids and gallstone disease

M. ANGELICO and THE GREPCO GROUP*

Several indirect data support the concept of a link between the metabolism of plasma lipoproteins and the occurrence of gallstone disease. These include the fact that most biliary stones are made of cholesterol; that lipoprotein lipids are the precursors of biliary lipids, including cholesterol and bile salts; and that the synthesis, uptake and degradation of plasma lipoproteins occur in the liver and may, therefore, influence the degree of bile cholesterol saturation.

There are, thus, good reasons to hypothesize that an abnormal lipoprotein metabolism in the liver may be a crucial event in relation to gallstone pathogenesis. However, despite the fact that a number of experimental and clinical studies have been devoted to this issue [1—4], the exact nature of the link between plasma lipoproteins and gallstone disease has not been clarified. Even in the largest clinical series, no definite association trends between serum lipids and gallstones have been found, except for a high frequency of gallstones in subjects with type IV hyperlipoproteinaemia [5]. During the last decade, the availability of gallbladder ultrasonography has allowed us to approach this contradictory problem from a novel point of view, i.e., the epidemiological one. I will now summarize the data obtained in this respect by the Rome group for Epidemiology and Prevention of Cholelithiasis (GREPCO). Part of these data were already presented 6 yr ago at this meeting [6], most of these have already been published [7].

Methods

Between January '81 and July '84 the GREPCO has enrolled 1244 men and 1081 women in a prospective ultrasonography-based survey of gallstone disease. Both men and women were civil servants working in Rome, who volunteered to participate in a generalized program of preventive medicine. The age range at time of enrollment was 20 to 64 yr in women and 20—69 yr

---

* For the composition of the GREPCO group see p. x (list of contributors).

L. Capocaccia et al. (eds), Recent advances in the epidemiology and prevention of gallstone disease, 121—127.
© 1991 *Kluwer Academic Publishers. Printed in the Netherlands.*

in men. The subject population included 65 cases with gallstones (G) and 37 cases with history of cholecystectomy (C) among males; 66 cases with G and 36 cases with C among females. A 6-yr prospective follow-up has already been completed in the female population. A total of 14 'new' cases of gallstones were detected from among 670 women who were re-examined by ultrasonography, which gives an incidence rate of 0.35% per year.

In brief, all subjects enrolled underwent gallbladder ultrasonography, a physical examination and completed a precoded questionnaire. Fasting plasma lipids and glucose were measured at entry, using conventional methods [8]. The statistical association of gallstone disease with the biochemical data and with the other variables measured were first analyzed by simple univariate analysis, after age standardization of the data. The associations were then reassessed using multiple regression analysis [9], to control for the role of possible confounders and ascertain their consistency and independency. Second-order interactions and quadratic terms were also considered to detect non-linear associations and interactions between variables.

Results and discussion

Univariate analysis

The average age-standardized serum lipids are given in Table 1. The data for serum triglycerides were log-transformed, because of the wide distribution. Mean serum triglycerides were higher in both men and women with G and with a history of C than in those without G. This difference was statistically significant only in men. These results are in agreeement with previous reports in selected populations [5, 10].

Table 1. Age-standardized mean (± SD) levels of serum lipids in the GREPCO populations.

	Men (1239)			Women (1081)		
	G–F	G	C	G–F	G	C
Log-triglycerides (mg dl^{-1})	4.8 ± 0.7	5.0 ± 0.8[a]	4.9 ± 0.5	4.4 ± 0.3	4.5 ± 0.6	4.3 ± 0.6
Total cholesterol (mg dl^{-1})	217 ± 44	209 ± 44[b]	210 ± 80	206 ± 40	203 ± 37	205 ± 45
HDL-Cholesterol (mg dl^{-1})	44 ± 11	39 ± 12	44 ± 9	57 ± 11	53 ± 15	56 ± 9

[a] p < 0.05, statistically different from gallstone-free subjects.
[b] p < 0.001, statistically different from gallstone-free subjects.
G–F = Gallstone-free.
G = Presence of gallstones.
C = History of Cholecystectomy.

Total and LDL-cholesterol were slightly and not significantly lower in men and women with G than in those without G or with a history of C. HDL-cholesterol was significantly lower in men with G than in those without G or with a history of C. A similar, although not significant, trend was apparent among women.

Multivariate analysis

When the data were examined by multiple regression analysis, a pattern of plasma lipid-gallstone association, partially different from that observed at univariate analysis, emerged. In setting the proper multiple logistic regression models, we took into account the factors listed in Table 2. These include the putative risk factors for gallstones and, in addition, several inter-related

Table 2. List of variables inluded in the multiple logistic regression model.

Age
Body mass index
Physical activity
Family history of gallstone disease
History of weight reduction
Smoking habits
Use of hypolipidemic drugs
Alcohol consumption
Dietary intake of butter, olive oil and polyunsaturated fats
Age at menopause
Number of pregnancies
Use of oral contraceptives

Table 3. Factors statistically associated with the presence of gallstones: Results from a multiple logistic regression analysis[b].

	Men			Women	
Factor	Coefficient[a]	p value	Factor	Coefficient[a]	p value
Age	5.06	< 0.001	Age	4.68	< 0.001
Triglycerides	2.61	< 0.01	Triglycerides	2.73	< 0.01
Triglycerides × age	−2.29	< 0.05	(Cholesterol)	−2.49	< 0.05
			Body mass index	2.35	< 0.05
			Parity	2.78	< 0.01
			Parity × age	−2.56	< 0.05

[a] Standardized logistic coefficient.
[b] Last equation of the stepwise procedure.

variables and other possible confounders. The final equation resulting from a multivariate stepwise procedure is shown in Table 3, where only those factors significantly associated with the presence of gallstones in the gallbladder are shown, with their respective standardized logistic coefficients, in men and women, respectively.

In men, only two conditions were significantly associated with the presence of gallstones, i.e., increasing age and increasing triglycerides. These two factors were inversely interrelated, indicating that the relative risk of gallstones attributable to high plasma triglycerides is greater in younger than in older men. A similar inverse age-triglycerides interaction has also been reported in a recent case-control study [11]. In women, five factors were significantly associated with the presence of gallstones: these included three non-lipid factors, i.e., increasing age, body mass index (BMI) and the number of pregnancies, and two lipid factors, i.e., increasing triglycerides and decreasing total (or LDL) cholesterol. Square transformation of the cholesterol data was necessary to detect this latter association, which, as shown in Fig. 1, was curvilinear in shape. In other words, the probability of having gallstones increased linearly with an increase in plasma triglycerides, both in men and women, while it decreased with increasing plasma cholesterol levels in women.

When a history of cholecystectomy was taken as the dependent variable in the multivariate analysis, most of the above associations with serum lipids disappeared, except, in women, that with plasma triglycerides. This suggests that either cholecystectomy modifies the levels of serum lipids or that, less likely, subjects undergoing cholecystectomy have different lipid patterns than those who do not. In any case, these results clearly indicate that subjects with

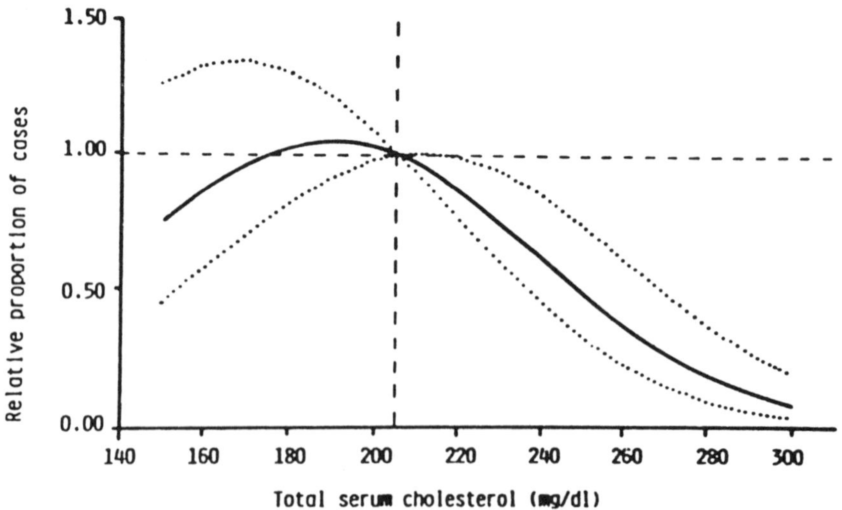

Fig. 1. Relationship of total serum cholesterol to the relative risk of gallstones in women.

a history of cholecystectomy cannot be regarded as representative of the whole spectrum of subjects with gallstone disease.

Prospective data

The associations between serum lipids and gallstones detected at univariate and multivariate analyses not only do not allow to address the first question, i.e., whether a defective lipoprotein metabolism is a determinant of gallstone disease, they also raise additional possibilities, including that gallstone disease may be itself responsible for a defective lipoprotein metabolism or, alternatively, that gallstones and lipoprotein abnormalities may be two expressions of a common (lipid) disorder. Only well-designed large prospective studies may address these questions. The preliminary data of the prospective follow-up already completed in 670 women, however, gives us some clues which may be worth presenting here. In this study, 14 incident cases of gallstones were found after a 6-yr follow-up. Table 4 shows the mean, age-standardized, levels of serum lipids in women who formed 'new' gallstones as compared to those who remained gallstone-free. A significantly ($p < 0.005$) higher mean triglyceride concentration was found in gallstone formers. When we looked at these data by multivariate analysis, taking into account age, body mass index, physical activity, parity, fasting glucose and other lipids, the only variable significantly predicting the formation of 'new' gallstones was the level of serum triglycerides. It is interesting to note that the predicting contribution of triglycerides completely obscured that of overweight and that a significant interrelation was found between the levels of serum triglycerides and the consumption of 'pasta' in our population.

Table 4. Age-standardized mean ($\pm$ SD) serum lipids measured at entry in 760 women who underwent a second gallbladder ultrasonography after a 6-yr follow-up.

	'New' gallstone formers (n = 14)	Gallstone-free (n = 746)
Triglycerides (mg dl^{-1})	114.3 $\pm$ 152.7[a]	84.1 $\pm$ 40.0
Total cholesterol (mg dl^{-1})	219.1 $\pm$ 34.4	202.8 $\pm$ 43.2
HDL-Cholesterol (mg dl^{-1})	53.8 $\pm$ 10.9	56.5 $\pm$ 11.2

[a] $p < 0.005$.

What do we learn from these epidemiological, cross-sectional and prospective data? Perhaps we may try to answer the earlier questions: is an abnormal lipoprotein metabolism a determinant of gallstone disease? We believe that the answer is 'probably yes'; is gallstone disease responsible for a defective lipoprotein metabolism? 'probably not'; are gallstones and lipoprotein abnormalities expressions of a common lipid disorder? 'most likely'. Epidemiological data on risk factors, if strength enough and prospectively validated, can be used to return back to pathophysiology and eventually stimulate interdisciplinary research. For example, the demonstration of an epidemiological positive association between gallstones and serum triglycerides, confirmed after prospective evaluation, at least in women, fits in with previous clinical and pathophysiological findings and also supports a lithogenic risk for type IV hyperlipoproteinaemia [5—10]. However, a number of queries remain unanswered. Hypertriglyceridaemia is a highly heterogeneous disorder, which may appear with multiple fenotypes and comprises inherited, acquired and transient conditions [11]. Are all these at risk for gallstones? Patients with type IV hyperlipoproteinaemia often have abnormalities in the synthesis, pool composition and enterohepatic dynamics of bile salts [12, 13], including deficient intestinal uptake [11]. Why is this so?, and how is this related to gallstones? Hypertriglyceridaemia may be due to chylomicron and VLDL overproduction in response to excess dietary substrates or increased apo-B synthesis, or to defective removal of triglyceride-rich lipoproteins [14]. Which of these mechanisms predispose to gallstones? Hypertriglyceridaemia is a physiological event in the postprandial period (which lasts one third of the day!). Does the degree and duration of postprandial lipemia influence gallstone formation?

We are now just entering the nineties, and we expect that, during the coming decade, the completion of major prospective epidemiological studies on gallstones disease, particularly the MICOL study, will provide enough data to clarify these points. However, without doubt, greater efforts from complimentary disciplines will also be of much help.

References

1. Schwartz CC, Halloran LG, Vlahcevic ZR, Gregory DH, Swell L (1978): Preferential utilization of free cholesterol from high density lipoprotein for biliary cholesterol secretion in man. *Science* 200: 62.
2. Thornton JR, Heaton KW, McFarlane DG (1981): A relation between high density lipoprotein cholesterol and bile cholesterol saturation. *Br Med J* 283: 1352—1354.
3. Ahlberg J, Angelin B, Einarsson K, Hellström K, Leijd B (1980): Biliary lipid composition in normo-and hyperlipoproteinaemia. *Gastroenterology* 79: 90—94.
4. Petitti DB, Friedman GD, Klatsky AL (1981): Association of a history of gallbladder disease with a reduced concentration of high density lipoprotein cholesterol. *N Engl J Med* 304: 1396—1398.
5. Ahlberg J, Angelin B, Einarsson K, Hellström L, Leijd B (1979): Prevalence of gallbladder disease in hyperlipoproteinaemia. *Dig Dis Sci* 24: 459.
6. M. Angelico and the GREPCO Group (1984): Relationships between serum lipids and cholelithiasis: observations in the GREPCO study, pp. 77—84 in: Capocaccia L, Ricci G, Angelico F, Angelico M, Attili AF (eds), *Epidemiology and Prevention of Gallstone Disease*, MTP Press, Lancaster and Boston.

7. The Rome Group for Epidemiology and Prevention of Cholelithiasis (GREPCO) (1988): The epidemiology of gallstone disease in Rome, Italy. Part II. Factors associated with the disease. *Hepatology* 8: 907—913.

8. Manual of Laboratory Operations, Lipid Research Clinic Programme (1974): DHEW Publ N (NIH) 75—328, Vol 1, p. 56.

9. BMDP Statistical Software (1981): Department of Biomathematics. University of California, Los Angeles, University of California Press.

10. Kadziolka R, Nilsson S, Schersten T (1977): Prevalence of hyperlipoproteinaemia in men with gallstone disease. *Scand J Gastroenterol* 12: 353.

11. Scragg RKR, Calvert GD, Oliver JR (1984): Plasma lipids and insulin in gallstone disease: a case control study. *Br Med J* 288: 1113—1119.

12. Angelin B, Herson KS, Brunzell JD (1987): Bile acid metabolism in hereditary forms of hypertriglyceridaemia: Evidence for an increased synthesis rate in monogenic familial hypertriglyceridaemia. *Proc Natl Acad Sci USA* 84: 5434—5438.

13. Angelin B, Einarsson L, Hellstrom K, Kallner M (1976): Elimination of cholesterol in hyperlipoproteinaemia. *Clin Sci Molec Med* 51: 393—397.

14. Angelin B, Einarsson K, Leijd B (1981): Bile acids and triglycerides metabolism in man, pp. 225—232 in: Paumgartner G, Stiehl A, Gerok W (eds), *Bile Acids and Lipids* Lancaster, England, MTP Press.

18. Dietary habits and gallstones: a study of male self-defense officials in Japan

S. KONO, N. IKEDA, F. YANAI, M. YAMAMOTO, K. SHINCHI and
K. IMANISHI

Introduction

Gallstones are less prevalent in Japan than in western countries [1—3].
Nevertheless, a changing pattern has been noted with respect to types of
gallstones in this country over the past decades. In Japan, pigment stones
used to be a predominant type of gallstones until the early 1950s, but
cholesterol stones have become more frequent [4–7]. In the 1970s, cholesterol stones accounted for about 80% of surgically removed stones [6, 7].
Since cholesterol gallstones are highly prevalent in western societies, the
change of gallstone composition observed in Japan has been generally
ascribed to westernization of Japanese diet [4, 7]. But this hypothesis remains
to be substantiated in the study of individuals [8].

Utilizing medical information derived from the retirement health examination program of the Self-Defense Forces (SDF) Fukuoka Hospital, we are
proceeding with a study on life style and diseases in male self-denfense
officials [9]. This report examined the relation of gallstone risk to the
consumption of selected foods and beverages, some of which could represent
typical Japanese and western dietary habits. The relation with other factors
such as cigarette smoking, alcohol drinking and obesity were also examined.

Materials and methods

In the retirement health examination program of the SDF Fukuoka Hospital,
free comprehensive medical examination has been offered for retiring
officials and employees of the SDF in northern Kyushu (including a part of
Yamaguchi Prefecture). The participation rate in this program is nearly
100%. For example, 98% of the retiring persons in the catchment areas
received the health examination in the period from April 1988 to March
1989. In October 1986, we included a questionnaire survey of life style in
the program for epidemiological study on life style and diseases. Women and
non-official employees were very few, and the study focused on male self-

L. Capocaccia et al. (eds), Recent advances in the epidemiology and prevention of gallstone disease, 129—137.
© 1991 Kluwer Academic Publishers. Printed in the Netherlands.

defense officials. The present study analyzed data accrued between October 1986 and December 1988.

The health examination was done during a 5-day admission from Monday to Friday and included abdominal ultrasonography (USG) as well as blood biochemical measurements and colonoscopy. The routine USG of the gallbladder was carried out with the subject overnight fast using a scanner equipped with a 3.5 MHz transducer (Aloka Co., Ltd, Japan). Repeated examination was done during the admission when the diagnosis was inconclusive. Based on the report of the USG study, the gallbladder status was classified into the following categories: gallstones, post-cholecystectomy state, gallbladder sludge, polyps, other disease conditions, normal gallbladder, and inconlusive. During the study period, a total of 1460 men aged 49—56 yr received the health examination. Results of the USG studies are summarized in Table 1.

Table 1. Results of ultrasonography of the gallbladder.

Gallbladder status	Number
Normal	1320
Gallstones	38
Post-cholecystectomy	22
Sludge	1
Polypoid lesions	68
Inconclusive	11
Total	1460

Self-administered questionnaires were distributed on the first day of admission and collected on the second day with supplementary interview for unfilled questions. The questionnaire inquired smoking and drinking habits, physical activities and dietary habits as well as family and personal medical history. Dietary questions asked both the frequency of consumption and amount consumed on average over the past one year for five non-alcoholic beverages (brewed coffee, instant coffee, black tea, green tea and milk), rice and soy bean paste soup. Only the frequency of consumption was asked regarding bread for breakfast, pickles, raw vegetables, fruits, raw fish, soy sauce cooked fish, broiled fish and meats. Precoded answers were used for the inquiry of consumption frequency, and the amount was answered by the conventional serving unit.

Smokers were defined as those who had ever smoked one cigarette or more over a period of one year or more. Ever-smokers were asked about average number of cigarettes smoked per day and years of smoking as well as whether they smoked currently. Questions on drinking habit demarcated never, past and current drinkers. Drinkers were defined as those who had ever drunk once per week or more during a period of one year or longer.

Those drinking currently answered to consumption frequency and amount consumed per occasion of five different beverages; *saké* (fermented product of rice), *shouchu* (distilled product of rice or other grains), beer, spirits (whiskey and brandy) and wine.

In the analysis, consumptions of foods and non-alcoholic beverages were categorized into three levels as shown in Table 2. Drinking black tea was too rare to justify the analysis. As for drinking habits, never and past drinkers were combined to minimize random fluctuation. There was little difference in gallstone risk between the two groups in a separate analysis. Alcohol intake was calculated from the reported frequencies and amounts of the five beverages using approximate concentrations of alcohol (*saké* 16%, *shouchu* 25%, beer 4.5%, spirits 40% and wine 12%).

Table 2. Category of the consumptions of foods and beverages in the comparison between gallstone cases and controls.

Food/dish	Low	Intermediate	High
Rice	< 3 bowls/day	3—4 bowls/day	⩾ 5 bowls/day
Soy bean paste soup	< 1 bowl/day	1 bowl/day	⩾ 2 bowls/day
Bread for breakfast	< once/week	1—5 times/week	daily
Pickles	< 4 times/week	4—5 times/week	daily
Raw vegetables	< 4 times/week	4—5 times/week	daily
Fruits	< 4 times/week	4—5 times/week	daily
Fish, combined[a]	< 4 times/week	4—5 times/week	daily
Meats	< 2 times/week	2—3 times/week	⩾ 4 times/week
Brewed coffee	< once/week	1—5 times/week	daily
Instant coffee	< 1 cup/day	1—2 cups/day	⩾ 3 cups/day
Green tea	< 3 cups/day	3—4 cups/day	⩾ 5 cups/day
Milk	< once/week	1—5 times/week	daily

[a] Consumptions of raw, soy sauce-cooked, and broiled fish were combined.

Body mass index, the weight in kilograms divided by the squared height in meters, was used as a measure of obesity. The SDF rank and history of gastrectomy were also examined in relation to the risk of gallstones. Reported history of gastrectomy completely agreed with that recorded by physicians, and gastrectomy within the past two years was not counted in the analysis.

Because the present study was cross-sectional, those with diseases which were considered to influence current dietary habits were excluded from the analysis. Excluding 2 men with post-operative cancer, 1 with Crohn's disease and 49 men with diabetes mellitus under dietary treatment among 1320 of normal gallbladder, comparisons were made between 38 men with gallstones and 1268 controls. Statistical analysis was done by logistic regression analysis in both univariate and multivariate analyses. Odds ratios were antilogarithms of regression coefficients of the corresponding indicator terms, and their 95% confidence intervals were calculated by using standard errors of the regression coefficients. Trends of the associations were assessed by assigning scores 0, 1 and 2 to the three levels of variables. P-values (two-sided) were based on ratios of regression coefficients to their standard errors. All statistical analyses were performed by the Statistical Analysis System (SAS) [10].

Results

Because ages of the study subjects were limited to narrow ranges in both gallstone cases and controls, age was not taken into consideration in the analysis. Mean ages were 52 years in the two groups, and ranges were 51—55 and 49—55 for the cases and controls, respectively.

Table 3 summarizes the associations of the consumptions of foods and non-alcoholic beverages with the risk of gallstones. Among 12 foods and beverages examined, only bread for breakfast was associated with an increased risk of gallstones showing a dose-response relationship. The elevated risk among those eating bread daily was statistically significant ($p =$ 0.02). Although men drinking instant coffee daily had an increased risk, there was no gradient increase in gallstone risk with increasing consumption of this beverage.

Table 4 shows the relation between non-dietary factors and gallstone risk. Prevalence of gallstones was significantly increased among men at the high

Table 3. Crude odds ratios (and numbers of gallstone cases/controls) according to consumption levels of foods and beverages.

Food/beverage	Consumption level[a]			P-value for trend
	Low	Intermediate	High	
Rice	1.0 (6/252)	1.3 (24/756)	1.3 (8/260)	0.66
Soy bean paste soup	1.0 (7/305)	1.6 (25/663)	0.9 (6/300)	0.84
Bread for breakfast	1.0 (13/625)	1.5 (13/427)	2.7 (12/216)	0.02
Pickles	1.0 (7/283)	1.5 (5/137)	1.2 (26/848)	0.69
Raw vegetables	1.0 (5/217)	1.5 (8/227)	1.3 (25/824)	0.71
Fruits	1.0 (13/520)	1.7 (11/256)	1.1 (14/492)	0.74
Fish, combined	1.0 (15/371)	0.7 (11/408)	0.6 (12/489)	0.20
Meats	1.0 (12/438)	1.2 (21/624)	0.9 (5/206)	0.99
Brewed coffee	1.0 (26/853)	1.3 (8/205)	0.6 (4/210)	0.57
Instant coffee	1.0 (13/641)	2.0 (12/292)	1.9 (13/335)	0.09
Green tea	1.0 (10/278)	0.8 (13/477)	0.8 (15/513)	0.67
Milk	1.0 (5/198)	1.5 (23/589)	0.8 (10/481)	0.42

[a] Same as the category in Table 2.

Table 4. Gallstone risk by the Self-Defense Forces (SDF) rank, history of gastrectomy, cigarette smoking and alcohol drinking.

Category	Number		Crude odds ratio (95% CI)
	Gallstone	Control	
SDF rank			
Low	28	1122	1.0
High	10	146	2.7 (1.3—5.8)
Prior gastrectomy			
(−)	34	1247	1.0
(+)	4	21	7.0 (2.3—21.5)
Cigarette-years[a]			
< 400	17	505	1.0
400—799	11	516	0.6 (0.3—1.4)
≥ 800	10	247	1.2 (0.5—2.7)
			Trend p = 0.88
Alcohol (mL day^{-1})			
0[b]	12	235	1.0
1—49	21	739	0.6 (0.3—1.1)
≥ 50	5	294	0.3 (0.1—1.0)
			Trend p = 0.03

[a] Cigarettes smoked per day multiplied by years of smoking.
[b] Never and past drinkers were combined.

Table 5. Crude odds ratios (and numbers of cases) for gallstones and post-cholecystecyomy state by body mass index[a].

Body mass index (kg m^{-2})	Gallstone	Post-cholecystectomy	Combined
< 22.5	1.0 (11)	1.0 (2)	1.0 (13)
22.5—24.9	1.5 (19)	4.8 (11)	2.0 (30)
≥ 25.0	1.0 (8)	6.4 (9)	1.9 (17)
Trend	P = 0.84	P = 0.01	P = 0.09

[a] Numbers of controls were 445, 510 and 313 for the low, intermediate and high levels of body mass index, respectively.

SDF ranks (major or above) and among those with a history of gastrectomy. While cigarette smoking was not related to the risk of gallstones, alcohol drinking was inversely related to gallstone risk. Because there was no clear association between prevalent gallstones and body mass index, we further examined the association with post-cholecystectomy state. Although the number was small, as shown in Table 5, post-cholecystectomy state was strongly associated with body mass index.

In order to evaluate whether eating bread for breakfast and alcohol drinking were associated with the risk of gallstones independently of each other and also of both the SDF rank and the history of gastrectomy, these four variables were simultaneously examined by multiple logistic regression models. As shown in Table 6, although none of the odds ratios was significantly deviated from unity with respect to eating bread for breakfast and alcohol drinking, the relations with these two variables did not much differed from those observed in the univariate analyses.

Table 6. Adjusted risk of gallstones according to the consumption levels of alcohol and bread for breakfast.[a]

Variable	Category	Adjusted odds ratio (95% CI)
Bread for breakfast	< once/week	1.0
	1—5 times/week	1.3 (0.6—3.0)
	daily	2.2 (0.9—5.1)
		Trend p = 0.08
Alcohol (mL day^{-})	0[b]	1.0
	1—49	0.6 (0.3—1.3)
	⩾ 50	0.4 (0.1—1.2)
		Trend p = 0.08

[a] Adjusted for the SDF rank, history of gastrectomy and either of the variables listed.
[b] Never and past drinkers were combined.

Discussion

The present population had a fairly low prevalence of gallstones with an overall rate of 4.1% including prior cholecystectomy (60/1449). This figure is slightly higher than observed in an earlier series of retiring self-dense men between 1978 and 1984 (2.9%) [3], but far lower than the rates reported in middle-aged men in western countries [11—13]. Risk factors of cholesterol gallstones had been mostly studied in high risk populations. Thus the study in a low risk population would be of some value in evaluating risk factors of this disease.

Studies based on health examination programs generally suffer from bias due to low participation rates, but the present study was free from such bias because of the almost complete participation. Weaknesses are, however, recognized in this study. Inherent drawbacks of cross-sectional study should be considered in interpreting the findings. Current dietary habits may be irrelevant to the formation of gallstones because a number of years are required for stones to become a detectable size [14]. We must assume that dietary habits at the age of early 50s have not changed much over the past few decades. Further, self-defense officials are not representative of the general population of Japanese men, and the findings of the present study may not be generalized.

Accuracy in dietary assessment is another problem in this type of study. We have not validated the dietary questions used in the present study, yet some of the items were found to have a high reproducibility. Table 7 shows the results of reproducibility study which was carried out on 49 males receiving the retirement health examination in January of 1989 with an interval of 1—2 months. We have used a slightly modified questionnaire since the beginning of 1989, but the dietary questions are essentially the same as those of the former questionnaire. It should be noted that reproducibility of bread for breakfast was much better than alcohol drinking.

Table 7. Reproducibility of dietary assessment in 49 male self-defense officials with an interval of 1—2 months.

Food/beverage	Intraclass correlation coefficient[a]
Rice	0.44
Soy bean paste soup	0.67
Bread for breakfast	0.78
Pickles	0.78
Raw vegetables	0.54
Fruits	0.44
Fish, combined	0.70
Meats	0.37
Brewed coffee	0.69
Instant coffee	0.81
Green tea	0.55
Milk	0.80
Alcohol	0.61

[a] Based on the category of three levels described in Table 2.

Eating bread for breakfast is a typical western dietary habit while rice, soy bean paste soup and pickles are traditional Japanese foods. Because it is unlikely that the consumption of bread itself is associated with the risk of gallstones, the observed association with eating bread for breakfast is interpreted as a supportive evidence for the idea that westernized diet is responsible for the occurrence of cholesterol gallstones in Japan. The westernization of Japanese diet in the postwar decades has been empirically related to the concurrent change in the gallstone composition in Japan [4—7]. The present study enforced the link between westernized diet and cholesterol gallstones in this country.

The inverse relation between alcohol intake and gallstone risk is consistent with the previous observations in western populations [15—18]. A cross-sectional study of civil servants in Rome found no association with alcohol consumption [19]. In that study, five classes of daily wine consumption were scored, and mean scores were compared between those with and without gallstones. The lack of association may be due to inappropriate measurement of alcohol intake or to a possibly small variation of wine consumption in that population. The protective effect of moderate alcohol intake against gallstone formation is also supported by experimental studies. Alcohol intake was found to lower the bile cholesterol saturation in humans [20] and to inhibit the formation of gallstones in animals [21].

Obesity is a well known risk factor for cholesterol gallstones [8]. In this study, obesity as expressed by body mass index was not associated with prevalent gallstones, but this is not necessarily an incompatible finding when the nature of cross-sectional study is considered. In fact, there was a strong association between body mass index and post-cholecystectomy state. If gallstones in obese men grow large enough to warrant cholecystectomy at earlier ages, then the association between obesity and prevalent gallstones would not emerge. Some of the previous studies have failed to find the association between obesity and gallstone disease in males and suggested possible differential effect of obesity between males and females [16, 19]. The present findings indicate that obesity plays an important role in the formation of gallstones in males as well. Regarding cigarette smoking, no appreciable association was found in the present study. Several studies have examined the relation between cigarette smoking and gallstone risk, but their findings are disparate [15, 17, 19, 22]. It is unlikely that cigarette smoking is an important factor in the formation of gallstones.

Gastrectomy has been suspected to be associated with an increased risk of gallstones [23, 24]. Although the increased risk among men who had undergone gastrectomy was substantial, it should be noted that such men were few. It is estimated that only 10% of gallstone cases are attributable to prior gastrectomy in the study population. Further study is needed to clarify specific dietary components responsible for the occurrence of cholesterol gallstones.

Acknowledgements

We are grateful to the nurses of the Second Ward of the Self-Defense Forces Fukuoka Hospital for their cooperation and to Ms. Taeko Shimoyama for her continuous efforts in handling collected data.

References

1. Brett M, Barker DJP (1976): The world distribution of gallstones. *Int J Epidemiol* 5: 335—41.

2. Nomura H, Kashiwagi S, Hayashi J, Kajiyama W, Ikematsu H, Noguchi A, Tani S, Goto M (1988): Prevalence of gallstone disease in a general population of Okinawa, Japan. *Am J Epidemiol* 128: 598—605.

3. Kono S, Kochi S, Ohyama S, Wakisaka A (1988): Gallstones, serum lipids, and glucose tolerance among male officials of Self-Defense Forces in Japan *Dig Dis Sci* 33: 839—44.

4. Kameda H (1964): Gallstone disease in Japan: a report of 812 cases. *Gastroenterology* 46: 109—14.

5. Nakayama F, Miyake H (1970): Changing state of gallstone disease in Japan. *Am J Surg* 120: 794—9.

6. Matsushiro T, Suzuki N, Sato T, Maki T (1977): Effects of diet on glucaric acid concentration in bile and the formation of calcium bilirubinate gallstones. *Gastroenterology* 72: 630—3.

7. Nagase M, Tanimura H, Setoyama M, Hikasa Y (1978): Present features of gallstones in Japan: a collective review of 2144 cases. *Am J Surg* 135: 788—90.

8. Bennion LJ, Grundy SM (1978): Risk factors for the development of cholelithiasis in man. *N Engl J Med* 299: 1161—7, 1221—7.

9. Kono S, Ikeda N, Yanai F, Yamamoto M, Shigematsu T (1990): Serum lipids and colorectal adenoma among male self-defense officials in northern Kyushu, Japan. *Int J Epidemiol* 19: 274—8.

10. Harrell FE, Jr. (1983): The LOGIST procedure, pp. 181—202 in: Joyner SP (ed), *SUGI Supplemental Library User's Guide*. Cary, North Carolina, SAS Institute Inc.

11. Rhomberg HP, Judmair G, Lochs A (1984): How common are gallstones? *Br Med J* 289: 1002.

12. Jørgensen T (1987): Prevalence of gallstones in a Danish population. *Am J Epidemiol* 126: 912—21.

13. The Rome Group for Epidemiology and Prevention of Cholelithiasis (GREPCO) (1988): The epidemiology of gallstone disease in Rome, Italy. Part I. Prevalence data in men. *Hepatology* 8: 904—6.

14. Mok HYI, Druffel ERM, Rampone WM (1986): Dating gallstones from atmospheric radiocarbon produced by nuclear bomb explosions. *N Engl J Med* 314: 1075—7.

15. Friedman GD, Kannel WB, Dawber TR (1966): The epidemiology of gallbladder disease: observations in the Framingham study. *J Chron Dis* 19: 273—92.

16. Scragg RKR, McMichael AJ, Baghurst PA (1984): Diet, alcohol, and relative weight in gallstone disease: a case-control study. *Br Med J* 288: 1113—9.

17. Diehl AK, Haffner SM, Hazuda HP, Stern MP (1987) Coronary risk factors and clinical gallbladder disease: an approach to the prevention of gallstones. *Am J Public Health* 77: 841—5.

18. Maclure KM, Hayes KC, Colditz GA, Stampfer MJ, Speizer FE, Willett WC (1989): Weight, diet, and the risk of symptomatic gallstones in middle-aged women. *N Engl J Med* 321: 563—9.

19. The Rome Group for Epidemiology and Prevention of Cholelithiasis (GREPCO) (1988): The epidemiology of gallstones in Rome, Italy. Part II. Factors associated with the disease. *Hepatology* 8: 907—13.

20. Thornton J, Symes C, Heaton K (1983): Moderate alcohol intake reduces bile cholesterol saturation and raises HDL cholesterol. *Lancet* ii: 819—22.

21. Schwesinger WH, Kurtin WE, Johnson R (1988): Alcohol protects against cholesterol gallstone formation. *Ann Surg* 207: 641—6.

22. Layde PM, Vessey MP, Yeates D (1982): Risk factors for gall-bladder disease: a cohort study of young women attending family planning clinics. *J Epidemiol Community Health* 36: 274—8.

23. Anderson JR, Ross AHM, Din NA, Small WP (1980): Cholelithiasis following peptic ulcer surgery: a prospective controlled study. *Br J Surg* 67: 618—20.

24. Lorusso D, Misciagna G, Noviello MR, Tarantino S (1988): Cholelithiasis after Billroth II gastric resection. *Surgery* 103: 579—83.

19. Gallbladder and pregnancy

A. MARINGHINI, M. CIAMBRA, P. BACCELLIERE, M. RAIMONDO,
R. GRASSO, M. RANDAZZO, A. ORLANDO, L. BARRESI,
S. SAMMARCO, F. TINÈ, D. GULLO, G. AGNELLO and
L. PAGLIARO

Introduction

Epidemiological studies throughout the world show that cholesterol gall-stones (GS) occur more commonly in women than in men [1].

We have recently demonstrated that biliary sludge (SL) is a common ultrasonographic (US) finding after delivery and usually spontaneously disappears in almost all patients in the first year of follow-up (Fig. 1) [2].

US is the most accurate tool for diagnosis of GS or SL [3, 4].

Aim of this study is to investigate prospectively the incidence of SL and GS in women during and after pregnancy, the predictive factors for their presence and their prevalence in a control group of women with or without Oral Contraceptive Use (OCU).

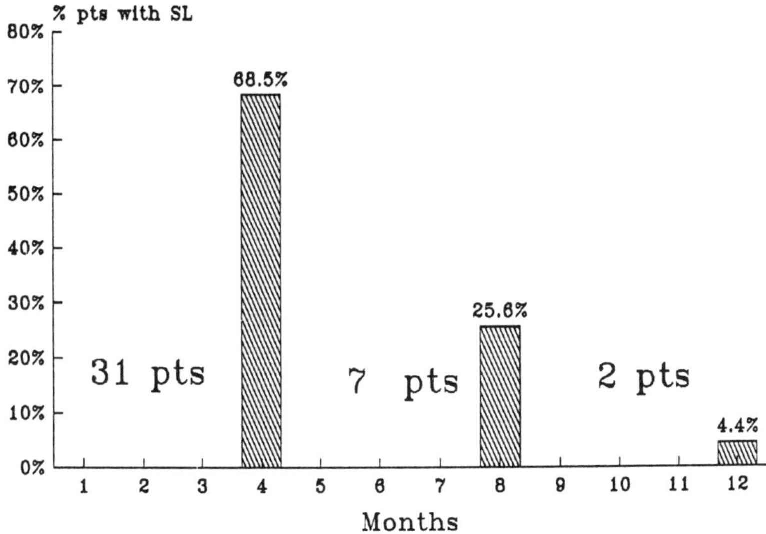

Fig. 1. SL in gallbladder after delivery.

L. Capocaccia et al. (eds), Recent advances in the epidemiology and prevention of gallstone disease, 139–145.
© 1991 *Kluwer Academic Publishers. Printed in the Netherlands.*

Patients and methods

All pregnant women admitted to the outpatient service of our hospital (Jan 86—Dec 87) were enrolled (n = 182, mean age 27.8 +/− 4.2 yr). All subjects observed during the same period for contraception were used as controls (n = 99, mean age 30.8 +/− 8.1 yr).

Pregnant women were submitted to US and clinical interview at the 3° and 6° month of pregnancy and 2—4 weeks after delivery. All controls were submitted to US and clinical interview, only once at presentation.

After an overnight fast the US examinations were always carried out using a high-resolution real-time scanner with a 3.5 MHz linear array transducer. The examinations were performed by two observers with the subjects supine, oblique with right side up, during the change from one position to another, and occasionally in the standing position.

All the patients were on a free diet, diagnosis of gallstones or sludge was considered if both observers were in agreement. The examiners performing ultrasonography were blind to each other's intepretations, and to previous examinations in pts during follow up.

Agreement between the observers was obtained for 97% of the patients (disagreement was registered only for SL). Three patients in pregnancy and one between controls were excluded because cholecystectomized. A diagnosis of SL was made when diffuse low-amplitude echoes forming a fluid-fluid level were present on US [4]. SL echoes were either heterogeneous with non-shadowing echogenic foci from 2 to 5 mm in size or homogeneous. When heterogeneous echoes were present, simple SL could not be differentiated from small stones which did not completely obstruct the US beam [3, 5]. Consequently, the diagnosis of GS was made when shadowing gravity dependent echogenic structures were observed in the gallbladder. To exclude slice-thickness artifact echoes that can mimic SL, we followed the suggestions of Goldstein and Madrazo [6].

Statistical analysis

Statistical significance was tested by Student's t-test for age, and by the Chi-square test (with Yates' correction when appropriate) for non-parametric data using the Statistical Package for Social Science (SPSS) [7, 8, 9]. The method of multiple logistic regression (using the Bio-Medical Data Processing, BMDP) was used to estimate the Odds Ratio, adjusted for the other variables in the model, for the presence of GS or SL versus normal.

The predictive factors for presence of GS or SL considered were age, obesity, months of previous use of oral contraceptives, number of previous pregnancies or deliveries.

Age and months of use of oral contraceptives were considered as continuous variables to increase the sensitivity of the model, 95% confidence limits for the Odds Ratio were obtained using Woolf's methods [7–9]. Obesity was defined as a body weight that exceeds the ideal body weight for age by 20% or more. (The ideal body weight was calculated utilizing acceptable weights as recommended by the Fogarty Conference, U.S.A. 1979 and the Royal College of Physicians, 1983) [10].

Cumulative incidence rate (and 95% confidence limits) of SL and GS in P was calculated by actuarial methods [11].

Results

In this paper we shall show preliminary data on 125 patients followed for all pregnancy, and 57 patients that are still in pregnancy at the first (n = 26) or at the second (n = 31) trimester. The first data on follow-up of women after delivery will be showed too.

We have enrolled 99 controls: we found SL in 7 and GS in 4 patients. Table 1 shows the relationship between the presence of GS and SL and the use of oral contraception.

Table 1. Relationship between Oral Contraceptive Use (OCU) and presence of SL and GS.

OCU (months)	N. pts	SL	GS
0	37	2 (5.4%)	1 (2.7%)
1—6	20	0	0
>6	42	5 (11.9%)	3 (7.14%)

Table 2. Predictive factors for presence of GS and SL.

	OR (Confidence limits 95%)
1. for GS	
— Pregnancy	12.27 (3.26—46.13)
— Age > 35 yr	8.41 (2.28—30.93)
2. for SL	
— Pregnancy	29.7 (12.6—70.2)

Follow-up studies during pregnancy demonstrated a cumulative incidence of SL in 14.3% of patients at the first trimester, 26.1% at the second and 41% after delivery (Fig. 2). We found GS in 15 patients at the first trimester and 6 new GS after delivery (Fig. 3).

We have followed up 9 patients with stones after delivery for 6 months: a

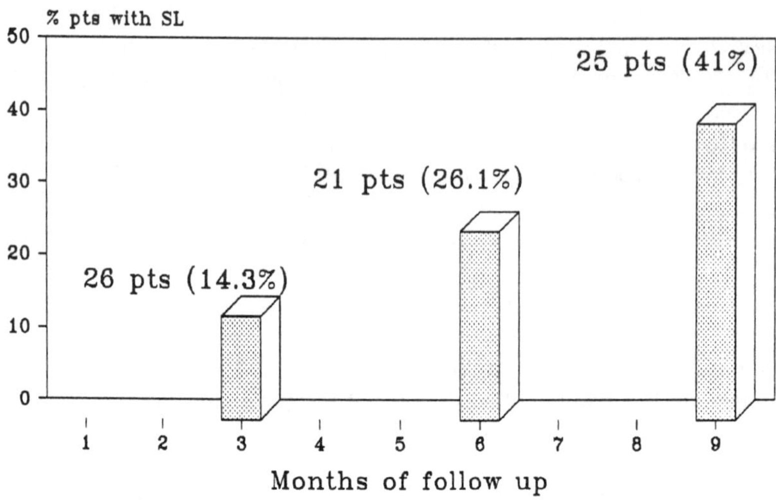

Fig. 2. Cumulative incidence of SL in 182 pts followed up during pregnancy (actuarial methods).

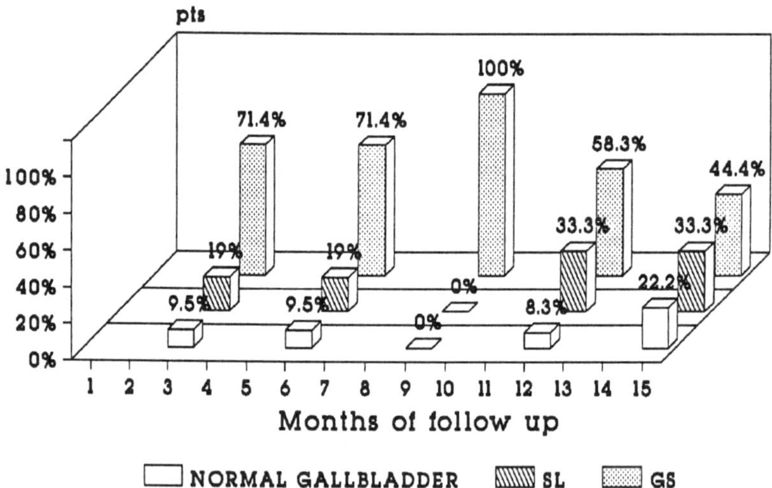

Fig. 3. US follow-up in pts with GS diagnosed during and/or after pregnancy.

spontaneous disappearance of GS was observed in 2, while 3 had only SL in gallbladder (Fig. 3).

Between the several analyzed predictive factors for presence of GS or SL, we found that age over 35 and pregnancy were significant for GS while only pregnancy was significant for presence of SL.

Discussion

Pregnancy is considered a major risk factor for cholesterol cholelithiasis, but no systematic study directly linking pregnancy to the presence of SL or GS has been performed.

In a recent study we found that a large number of women had SL in the gallbladder after delivery while a few patients had GS: after one year only 4.4% of patients with SL and 86.7% of patients with GS had abnormal US findings in the gallbladder (Fig. 1) [2].

In this paper we have showed preliminary data of a prospective study on gallbladder in pregnancy and in a control group.

We have confirmed a cumulative incidence of SL, after delivery, of 41% by actuarial methods. In the same period we found 6 new cases of stones.

Some of these stones spontaneously disappeared or became SL during the first months of follow up after delivery.

A prerequisite for cholesterol GS formation is the hepatic secretion of lithogenic bile [12—14]. In addition, major physicochemical changes, including nucleation [15], crystal formation and adherence of crystals [16—18], must occur in the gallbladder to generate cholesterol gallstones. Since these changes require time, retention of lithogenic bile in the gallbladder is necessary. If gallbladder emptying were prompt and complete, lithogenic bile and any cholesterol crystals that might have formed would pass into the duodenum promptly. GS therefore would not occur. During pregnancy both these prerequisites are present. In fact, during the last trimester of pregnancy changes in hepatic bile occur owing to high estrogen levels [19], while Everson et al. have demonstrated that pregnant women empty their gallbladders slowly [20]. They argue that during pregnancy, and particularly in the last trimester, lithogenic bile, in the presence of conspicuous gallbladder statis, may precipitate as cholesterol SL or GS.

We looked for SL in the gallbladders of our patients by US because it has been shown experimentally that pigment granules, calcium bicarbonate, cholesterol crystals and small stones were echogenic [4, 21].

Several epidemiological studies throughout the world have hypothized an association between GS and the female sex.

Bockus et al. in 1935 observed an elevated prevalence of cholesterol GS in women: the most of their symptomatic patients were found to be pregnant [22].

Friedman et al. in the Framingham study confirmed a marked female predominance of GS with an overall incidence rate about twice as high in women as in men [23].

Later autoptic, case control and large cohort studies have confirmed Bockus' statement about elevated prevalence of cholesterol GS in females [24—27].

This elevated female-to-male incidence ratio decreases slightly with increasing age and perists only during the childbearing year [23–27].

Conflicting results have been obtained on relationship between GS and pregnancy, but a critic review on literature seems to demonstrate that parity is associated with GS only in youngers [24, 28—31]. These results may be compared with an elevated prevalence of GS in youngers with oral contraceptive use suggested by two large case-control studies [29, 32] not confirmed in a recent Danish cohort study [30].

We have analyzed several risk factors for GS and/or SL presence. We found that only age over 35 and the presence of pregnancy were significant predictive factors for presence of GS while only pregnancy was demonstrated to be a predictive factor for SL presence. We failed to confirm other risk factors as obesity or others that seem to be related to GS [2, 24, 31, 33], but we have to wait for definitive data with a larger sample because 21 patients with GS may be not enough to point out some relationship.

In conclusion, we confirm that SL occurs frequently during and after pregnancy and we can add that also stones may appear and disappear during and after pregnancy.

References

1. Bennion LJ, Grundy SM (1978): Risk factors for the development of cholelithiasis in man. *N Engl J Med* 299: 1161—1167.
2. Maringhini A, Marcenò MP, Lanzarone F, et al. (1987): Sludge and stones in gallbladder after pregnancy. *J Hepatology* 5: 218—223.
3. Coopberg PL, Burhenne HJ (1980): Real-time ultrasonography. Diagnostic technique of choice in calcolous gallbladder disease. *N Engl J Med* 302: 1277—1279.
4. Conrad MR, Janes JO, Dietch Y (1979): Significance of low level echoes within the gallbladder. *Am J Roentgenol* 132: 967—972.
5. Taylor KJ, Jacobson P, Jaffe CR (1979): Lack of an acoustic shadow on scans of gallstones. A possible artifact. *Radiology* 131: 469—472.
6. Goldstein A, Madrazo B (1981): Slice thickness artifacts in gray-scale ultrasound. *J Clin Ultrasound* 9: 365—375.
7. Maxwell AE (1961): Analyzing Qualitative Data. London, Redwood Press Limited.
8. Dixon WJ, Brown MB, Englman L et al. (1979): Bio Medical Data Processing. Statistical Software. Berkeley, University of California Press.
9. Nye NY, Hull CH, Jenkins JG, Steinbrenner K, Bent DH (1975): Statistical Package Foe the Social Sciences. 2nd Edn. New York, Mc Graw — Hill Book Company.
10. Passmore R, Eastwood MA. 8th Edn. (1986): Human Nutrition and dietetics. p. 516, **Churchill Livingstone Edinburgh London Melbourne and New York.**
11. Cutler SJ and Ederer F (1958): Maximum utilization of the life table method an analyzing survival. *J Chronic Dis* 8: 659.
12. Small DM (Ingelfinger FJ, Ebert RB, Findlan DM, Realman AS (eds), (1974): Controversies in Internal Medicine II. Management of gallstones, particularly the silent variety: advantages of a varied and individual approach, p. 545 Philadelphia, Saunders.
13. Small DM (1980): Cholesterol nucleation and growth formation in gallstones formation. *N Engl J Med* 302: 1305—1306.

14. Shaffer A, Small DM (1976): Gallstones disease pathogenesis and management. *Curr Probl Surg* 13: 1—72.
15. Holan KR, Holzbach RT, Herman RE et al. (1979): Nucleation time: a key factor in the pathogenesis of cholesterol gallstone disease. *Gastroenterology* 77: 611—617.
16. Sedhagat A, Grundy SM (1980): Cholesterol crystals and the formation of cholesterol gallstones. *N Engl J Med* 302: 1274—1277.
17. Walton AG (1967): The Formation and the Properties of Precipitate. Vol. 23. New York, Intersciences.
18. Craven BM (1967): Crystal structure of cholesterol monohydrate. *Nature* 260: 727—729.
19. Lynn J, Williams L, O'Brien J et al. (1973): Effects of estrogen on bile. *Ann Surg* 178: 514—524.
20. Everson GT, McKimley C, Lawson M, Johnson M, Kern F Jr (1982): Gallbladder function in the human female: effect of the ovulatory cycle, pregnancy and contraceptive steroids. *Gastroenterology* 81: 711—719.
21. Glancy JJ, Goddard J, Pearson DE (1980): In vitro demonstration of cholesterol crystals' high echogenicity relative to protein particles. *J Clin Ultrasound* 8: 27—29.
22. Bockus HL, Willard JH, Metzerg HN (1935): Role of infection and of disturbed cholesterol metabolism in gallstone genesis. *Pa Med J* 39: 482.
23. Friedman GD, Kannel WB, Dawber TR et al. (1966): The epidemiology of gallbladder disease: observations in the Framingham study. *J Chronic Dis* 19: 273—292.
24. Barbara L, Sama C, Morselli Labate AM et al. (1987): A population study on the prevalence of gallstone disease: the Sirmione study. *Hepatology* 7: 913—917.
25. Rome group for the Epidemiology and Prevention of Cholelithiasis (GREPCO) (1988): The epidemiology of gallstone disease in Rome, Italy. Part I Prevalence data in men. *Hepatology* 8: 904—906.
26. Nomura H, Kashiwagi S, Hayashy J et al. (1989): Prevalence of gallstone disease in a general population of Okinawa, Japan. *Am J Epidemiol*
27. Mauer KM, Everhart JE, Ezzati TM et al. (1989): Prevalence of gallstone disease in Hispanic populations in the United States. *Gastroenterology* 96: 487—492.
28. Rome group for the Epidemiology and Prevention of Cholelithiasis (GREPCO) (1988): The epidemiology of gallstone disease in Rome, Italy. Part II. Factors associated with the disease. *Hepatology* 8: 907—913.
29. Scragg RKR, McMichael AJ, Seamark RF (1984): Oral contraceptives, pregnancy and endogenous oestrogen in gallstone disease: a case-control study. BMJ 288: 1795—1799.
30. Jorgensen T (1988): Gallstones in a Danish population: fertility period, pregnancies and exogenous female sex hormones. *Gut* 29: 433—439.
31. Maclure MK, Hayes KC, Graham A et al. (1989): Weight, diet, and the risk of symptomatic gallstones in middle-aged women. *N Engl J Med* 321: 563—569.
32. Royal College of General Practicioners Oral Contraception Study (1982): Oral contraceptives and gallbladder disease. *Lancet* ii: 957—959.
33. GREPCO (1984): Prevalence of gallstone disease in an Italian adult female population. *Am J Epidemiol* 119: 796—805.

20. Risk factors for gallstone disease: the Sirmione study

E. RODA, L. BARBARA, G. L. CORNIA, D. FESTI, R. FRABBONI,
A. M. MORSELLI LABATE, M. C. NACCHIERO, S. PARRO,
G. POLLINI, M. ROSSI, A. G. RUSTICALI, C. SAMA, F. TARONI,
G. TASSINARI, C. BANTERLE, S. COLASANTI, G. FORMENTINI,
O. MORENI, F. NARDIN, M. C. PILIA and A. PUCI

Introduction

Prevention of cholelithiasis, still at a very early stage, depends largely on a clear understanding of events concerning its pathogenesis and risk factors.

In the past many factors on clinical experiences or case-control studies (Table 1) have been considered capable of promoting gallstone development. However the current literature about epidemiology of gallstone make it very difficult to support clinical impression with statistics.

Table 1. Putative factors associated with the presence of cholesterol gallstones.

Ethnic	American Indians, Northern Europe, West > Orient
Age	
Sex	Women
	Pregnancy
Familial	
Weight	Obesity
	Rapid weight loss
Bile acid malabsorption	Distal ileal disease, resection or by-pass, cystic fibrosis
Drugs	Clofibrate
	Oral contraceptives
Diabetes	
Hyperlipidemias	
Diet	

Methods

We initiated in 1982 a longitudinal study on the incidence and risk factors of gallstone disease (GD) in the town of Sirmione [1].

As part of this ongoing study, factors associated with GD were identified during the first cross-sectional study in 1982.

L. Capocaccia et al. (eds), Recent advances in the epidemiology and prevention of gallstone disease, 147—152.
© 1991 *Kluwer Academic Publishers. Printed in the Netherlands.*

For this purpose our study protocol included a medical and family history, the measurement of height and weight, laboratory analysis of fasting blood samples (glucose, total and HDL cholesterol, triglycerides, AST, ALT, and GGT), and a questionnaire inquiring on the use of drugs (particularly estroprogestinic and cholesterol lowering agents).

Moreover, the daily intake of major nutrients (energy, proteins, total fats, cholesterol, carbohydrates, starch and total sugar, dietary fibre and alcohol) has been evaluated in the studied population with the method of dietary recall, by a term of 6 dietitians particularly trained in epidemiological studies.

In our study we have considered obese those subjects with a body mass index (BMI) greater than 30 kg m^{-2}.

In order to define hypertriglyceridemic and hypercholesterolemic subjects, the 70th sex and age specific percentile was chosen as cut-off point.

Subjects with a known history of diabetes or with fasting glucose levels higher than 140 mg dl^{-1} have been considered diabetic in our study.

Results

Age and female sex were found to be associated with an increased prevalence of gallstone disease [2]. Among the other possible associated factors we found an increased prevalence of gallstone disease in subjects who were obese at the time of the study in comparison to non-obese subjects (Age and sex standardized Mantel-Haenszel Relative Risk [3]: RR_{MH} = 1.66; 95% c.l. = 1.22 to 2.25). Prevalence was higher also in subjects who have been obese in the past, although not statistically significant (Fig. 1).

In our population 41 subjects were defined diabetic according to our criteria; we failed to observe an association between diabetes and gallstone disease (RR_{MH} = 1.12; 95% c.l. = 0.57 to 2.21) (Fig. 1).

Hypercholesterolemic subjects did not show an increased frequency of gallstones (RR_{MH} = 1.10; 95% c.l. = 0.84 to 1.46); however an association between hypertriglyceridemia and gallstone disease has been observed (RR_{MH} = 1.65; 95% c.l. = 1.27 to 2.13) (Fig. 2).

Parity has been shown to be associated with gallstone disease (Age standardized RR_{MH} = 1.60; 95% c.l. = 1 to 2.57), and relative risk increased with the number of pregnancies, particularly in young women (Fig. 3). The frequency of gallstone disease in women who ever used, and in those who never used, estroprogestinic drugs was not significantly different (RR_{MH} = 0.76; 95% c.l. = 0.46 to 1.25).

As far as the dietary habit is concerned, we did not found a difference in the daily intake of major nutrients in subjects with or without gallstones (Fig. 4). Gallstone subjects, older than 40 yr, had a significantly (P < 0.01; ANOVA adjusted for sex) lower fiber intake (361 ± 134 mg kg^{-1} BW day^{-1}; mean ±SD) in comparison to non gallstone subjects (408 ± 160 mg kg^{-1} BW day^{-1}). Alcohol consumption was significantly lower (P < 0.05;

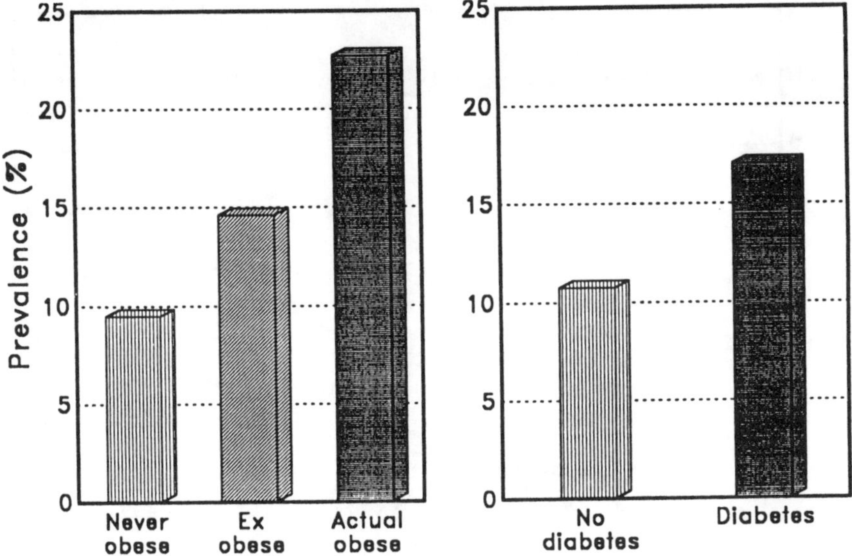

Fig. 1. Prevalence of gallstone disease in relation to obesity and diabetes. Subjects who were obese at the time of the study had a significantly higher (see text) frequency of gallstone than non obese subjects. No significant increase was found in subjects with diabetes.

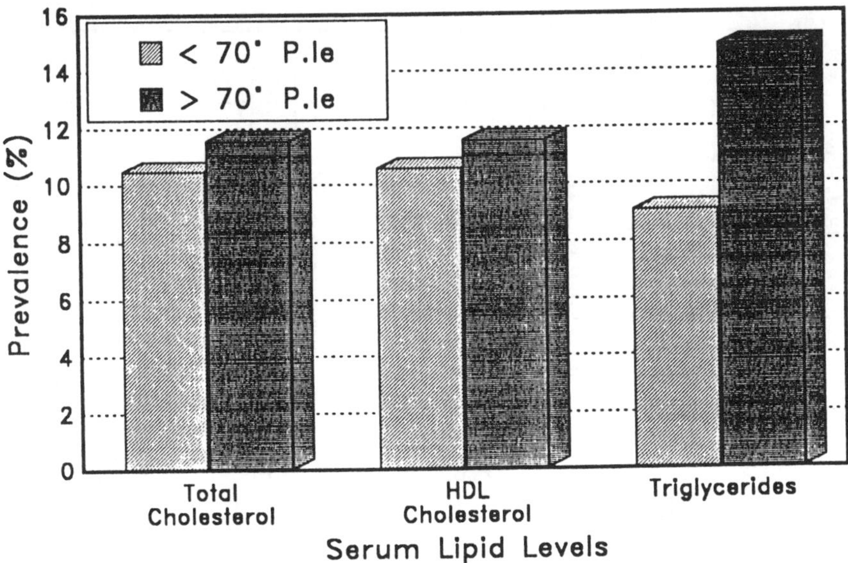

Fig. 2. Prevalence of gallstone disease in subjects with low and high levels of serum total and HDL cholesterol and triglycerides. The 70th sex and age specific percentile was chosen as cutoff point for defining risk. Subjects with high serum triglyceride levels had a significantly higher frequency of gallstone disease (see text).

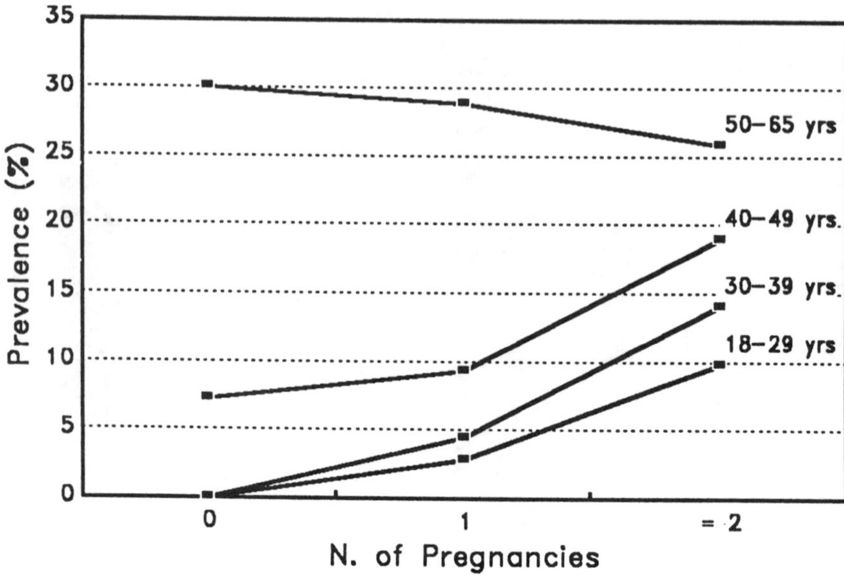

Fig. 3. Prevalence of gallstone disease in relation to the number of pregnancies. Prevalence increases significantly (see text) with the number of pregnancies in women younger than 50 yr.

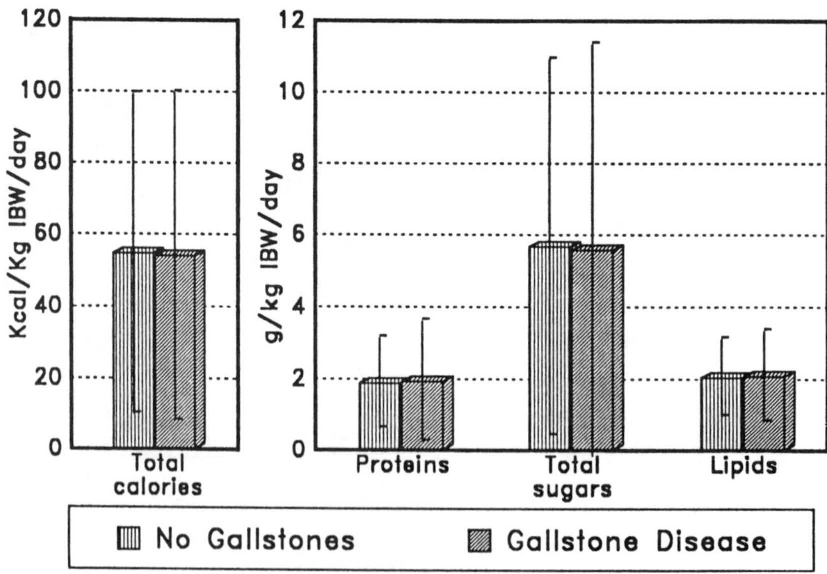

Fig. 4. Daily intake of major nutrients in 1982. No significant differences were observed between subjects with and without gallstones.

ANOVA adjusted for sex and age) in gallstone (36.2 $\pm$ 40.1 g day^{-1}) than in non gallstone subjects (48.5 $\pm$ 50.3 g day^{-1}).

Eighty-two percent (1325/1628) of the gallstone-free subjects who participated in the first study were reexamined in 1987 with the purpose of defining incidence and risk factors for gallstone disease. The incidence rate was significantly higher in the age span 40—65 yr (4.7%) than in younger subjects (1.2%) (P < 0.001; X^2 test). Incidence was not significantly different in males (3.4%) and females (2.7%). Obesity was associated with an increased incidence of gallstone disease (7.2% versus 2.7% in non-obese; RR_{MH} = 2.66; 95% c.l. = 1.23 to 5.77). Parity was also associated with a higher incidence of gallstone disease (3.2% in ever pregnant versus 0.7% in never pregnant), although not statistically significant (RR_{MH} = 4.50; 95% c.l. = 0.75 to 28.05). High serum triglyceride levels were not confirmed as a risk factor for gallstone disease. No difference in dietary habit has been observed between gallstone and non gallstone cases as far as energy, proteins, total fats, carbohydrates, starch, and total sugar are concerned. The daily intake of vegetable fibre was significantly lower in gallstone than in non-gallstone cases (96 $\pm$ 48 versus 115 $\pm$ 54 mg kg^{-1} BW day^{-1}; mean $\pm$ SD; P < 0.05); this is mainly due to the lower fibre intake observed in older (40—65 yr) gallstone patients (89 $\pm$ 46 mg kg^{-1} BW day^{-1}). Also the daily intake of cholesterol was significantly lower in gallstone than in non-gallstone cases (7.4 $\pm$ 2.5 versus 8.5 $\pm$ 3.0 mg kg^{-1} BW day^{-1}; P < 0.05).

Conclusion

In the Sirmione study during the first cross-sectional screening some factors were found to be associated with gallstone disease. They are: female sex, increasing age, obesity, parity and hypertriglyceridemia. Because relative risk estimates in prevalence studies may be biased since it is impossible to tell if a 'putative' factor arose before or after the disease, these data needed to be confirmed by the incidence study. At the moment, data on the 5-yr incidence are available, concerning 40 new cases of gallstone disease.

In spite of the limitation due to the small number of cases, age and obesity were confirmed as true risk factors for gallstone development. Some diet-related factors, as low fibre consumption, seem to be related to a higher incidence of gallstone disease.

References

1.   Barbara L, Sama C, Morselli Labate AM, Taroni F, Rusticali AG, Festi D, Sapio C, Roda E, Banterle C, Puci A, Formentini F, Colasanti S, and Nardin F (1987): A population study on the prevalence of gallstone disease: The Sirmione Study. *Hepatology* 7: 913—917.

2.   Festi D, Barbara L, Frabboni R, Morselli Labate AM, Nacchiero MC, Parro S, Pollini G, Roda E, Rossi M, Rusticali AG, Sama C, Taroni F, Tassinari G, Banterle C, Colasanti S, Formentini G, Moreni O, Nardin F, Pilia MC, Puci A (1990): Prevalence and incidence of gallstone disease: the Sirmione study. In: *Recent Advances in the Epidemiology and Prevention of Gallstone Disease* (in the same book).
3.   Mantel N, Haenszel W (1959): Statistical aspects of the analysis of data from retrospective studies of disease. *J Natl Cancer Inst* 22, 719—748.

21. Gallstones that form during rapid weight loss

L. J. SCHOENFIELD, P. H. BROOMFIELD, G. G. BONORRIS and
J. W. MARKS

Cholesterol gallstones can form during rapid loss of weight [1, 2]. Ursodeoxycholic acid (UDCA) decreases the biliary saturation index (SI) [3] while
aspirin (ASA) decreases biliary glycoproteins (GP) [4]. Therefore, UDCA or
ASA might prevent the formation of gallstones that depends upon increased
biliary saturation or glycoproteins, respectively. The aim of this study, as
previously reported [5], was to determine the effects of loss of weight during
administration of UDCA, ASA, or placebo on the biliary SI, glycoproteins,
cholesterol crystals, and gallstones.

Methods

Sixty-eight obese persons without gallstones were acceded to this study just
prior to their entering a program to lose weight on a diet of 520 kCal day^{-1}.
They were allocated randomly to receive, in double-masked fashion, capsules
of UDCA (U) 1200 mg day^{-1}, ASA (A) 1300 mg day^{-1}, or placebo (P).
These subjects were treated for 16 weeks or for less time if they reached
their goal-weight (average loss was 22 kg), developed gallstones, or left the
program sooner.

At baseline and after 4 weeks, ultrasonography was done to detect
gallstones and duodenal drainage was done for cholesterol crystals, biliary SI,
and glycoproteins (photometry). Three weeks after the capsules were
stopped, ultrasonography and duodenal drainage were done a final time.

Results

By 16 weeks, with placebo, cholesterol crystals formed in 6 patients and
gallstones in 5 whereas with UDCA no patients developed crystals or stones
(P < 0.05). With ASA, crystals were found in 1 patient and gallstones in the
only 2 patients who were non-compliant in taking their ASA.

The SI with placebo increased from 1.07 $\pm$ 0.26 to 1.29 $\pm$ 0.27 (P <

L. Capocaccia et al. (eds), Recent advances in the epidemiology and prevention of gallstone disease, 153—154.
© 1991 *Kluwer Academic Publishers. Printed in the Netherlands.*

0.001), with UDCA decreased from 1.11 ± 0.34 to 0.91 ± 0.24 (P < 0.001), and with ASA did not change significantly. With placebo, the glycoprotein increased 27.9 ± 14.5% (P < 0.001) but with UDCA or ASA did no change significantly.

The sequence of events in one untreated patient was increased biliary SI, arachidonate, prostagladin E2, and glycoprotein, then decreased nucleation time, and finally development of cholesterol crystals.

Conclusion

During weight loss in obese subjects, UDCA and possibly ASA, prevented biliary lithogenic changes and formation of gallstones.

References

1. Mok HYL, Bergman KV, Grundy SM (1979): Biliary lipid metabolism in obesity. Effects of bile acid feeding before and during weight reduction. *Gastroenterology* 76: 556—7.
2. Liddle RA, Goldstein RB, Saxton J (1989): Gallstone formation during weight-reduction dieting. *Arch Intern Med* 149: 1750—3.
3. Stiehl A, Raedsch R, Rudolph G, Walker S (1984): Effect of ursodeoxycholic acid on biliary bile acid and bile lipid composition in gallstone patients. *Hepatology* 4: 107—11.
4. Lee SP, Carey MC, LaMont JT (1981): Aspirin prevention of cholesterol gallstone formation in prairie dogs. *Science* 211: 1429—31.
5. Broomfield PH, Chopra R, Sheinbaum RC, Bonorris GG, Silverman A, Schoenfield LJ, Marks JW (1989): Effects of ursodeoxycholic acid and aspirin on the formation of lithogenic bile and gallstones during loss of weight. *N Engl J Med* 319: 1567—72.

22. Concluding remarks

J. STAMLER

In these closing remarks, I would like, before coming to the question of prevention, to touch on a number of methodological and conceptual issues. I do so, not as an expert on gallstones but, rather, trying to bring to bear thirty years or more of learning on chronic disease epidemiology. I hope that what is still a young field, i.e., the epidemiology of gallstones, may gain by this experience and thus avoid repeating mistakes made in the past.

As we saw in the course of this conference, in developed countries, with the exception of Japan — an interesting exception with regard to several chronic diseases — gallstone disease is a mass (common) not a rare disease. Prevalence rates are high. Though incidence rates appear to be low (1% yr), if we think in terms of tens of millions of people and take a long view, i.e., for the decades of the life span going from late young adulthood or early middle-age into older age, these rates are not so low.

To quote Rudolf Virchow, mass diseases are due to 'disturbances of human culture.' All my experience with non-infectious diseases — severe atherosclerosis and coronary heart disease, high blood pressure, various cancers, cirrhosis, chronic obstructive lung disease — had led me to believe that this is a basic guiding principle for all of us. Our task as epidemiologists is to find out what about our civilization has produced these disturbances and to unravel the specific exposures. This applies also to gallstone disease.

In this regard I would like to call attention to the writings of Thomas McKeown, from England, who has written two books and published a seminal article in *The Lancet* which I make compulsory reading for every medical student. McKeown's paper discusses the nature of medical research and its two foci. One focus, involving most medical research, is concerned with mechanisms. Exposures are assumed. Given the exposure, the question being explored is: what goes on in the human body that leads from the exposure to the disease, i.e., pathophysiologic pathogenetic mechanisms. There is little or no attention paid to the exposures. The other focus is on what McKeown calls the origins of disease, i.e., the mass exposures or life styles that are the causes of mass occurrence of disease. What is going on out there in the mass, in our species' mode of life, in successive historic periods,

L. Capocaccia et al. (eds), Recent advances in the epidemiology and prevention of gallstone disease, 155—161.
© 1991 *Kluwer Academic Publishers. Printed in the Netherlands.*

that produces the evolving mass disease patterns of different eras and sites. McKeown emphasizes that medical research is generally one-sided and biased in its approach to disease and tends to focus on mechanisms and to neglect origins, exposures, etiology. In epidemiology we are of course concerned first and foremost with these latter aspects. In regard to the mass occurrence of gallstones, I suggest that much more rigorous and vigorous work is needed on issues of exposure, the disturbances of human culture producing this epidemic.

With that in mind, I want to add that it was very exciting in the course of this meeting to see the first population-based incidence data on gallstone disease. But, I emphasize, this is just a beginning. Fourteen cases here, 33 cases there, only 5 yr of follow-up: these are small numbers and therefore treacherous. The confidence interval around every rate is very big, hence comparisons across groups are limited in meaning. Moreover, there is very little possibility of doing multivariate analyses soundly with such small numbers. What is needed is patience and further work on prospective follow-up — and then on analyses, with ten, fifteen, twenty years of follow-up. I, personally, am working in Chicago on 25-yr and 30-yr follow-up data from the People's Gas Company Study and the Western Electric Study. The Framingham Study has a wealth of data with 30-yr follow-up. It is not only a question of numbers. We have reason to believe from some of our data that certain relationships emerge not only because you get more numbers, but because certain exposures are required for certain lengths of time before relationships are clear. So I urge patience and persistence, and understanding from pertinent organizations — i.e., funding organizations — to ensure that long-term follow-up is pursued.

Next I would like to comment about the types of epidemiological studies we generally do, where the work on the epidemiology of gallstones fits in with regard to these, and where there seem to be limitations and lacks, and what might be done to overcome these. First of all we have cross-sectional and, within the cross-sectional mode, case-control type studies. Clearly these are already under way. Take, for example, the multicenter study in Italy — MICOL — which is a fascinating cross-sectional study, destined, I'm led to believe, to become a prospective study. One interesting aspect of the MICOL study is that it is not just a within-population study, but could also be termed a cross-population study, related to the fact that Italy is still a country of considerable contrasts. This I will come back to later.

Particularly fruitful in cardiovascular epidemiology, and to the best of my knowledge not yet developed in the gallstone field (in part because there is no end point related to gallstones permitting use of WHO mortality data), are international cross-population studies. In the course of this workshop it was mentioned that gallstones may be rare in certain economically developing countries or at least among certain strata of the populations of those countries. However, there apparently are no good data. In my mind the effort should be made to obtain these, as many puzzling questions could be illuminated by such data. Indeed, it has been said that if one takes cross-population data and within-population data, where the cross-population data are positive and the within-population data are not, particularly in relation to diet, believe the cross-population data. This may be regarded by some as heresy. My view is that both types of data — within-population and cross-population — are needed. When contradictions arise, the challenge is to figure out why this is so. Often the contradiction is not real but apparent and relates to methodology.

Moreover, not only are there no cross-sectional international data, particularly comparing populations from developing and industrialized countries, there also are no studies of migrants. What happens with gallstone disease when life styles change as a result of migration? As you probably know, in the breast cancer, colon cancer, and coronary research areas, cross-population studies involving the effects of migration have been fruitful in enlightening us about exposures and their etiologic significance. Perhaps the Italian MICOL study has the ability to identify northern Italians who migrated from the south, and to analyze changes in life style as Italians migrate from the economically poorer south to the industrialized richer north. If this capability exists, then MICOL is the only study of its type so far on migrants that I know of. I urge that a real effort be made to broaden research to include such topics.

Next I would like to make some comments on what I consider to be some key questions of methodology. The sophisticated discussion on the sonographic work and the reliability study within the MICOL project are particularly interesting. This is a valuable reliability study, particularly meaningful for me at present, given my connection with one of the big on-going trials in the United States, the so-called TOMHS study, involving six groups receiving, for 'mild' hypertension, nutritional-hygienic plus drug treatment (1 of 5 different active medications). We are doing echocardiographic work in this study and have assessed reliability across readers with startling results. We started with technician readers; reliability studies soon taught us that this was far from optimal. Then we worked with five cardiologists and again disagreements were considerable. As a consequence, we changed to readings by only two cardiologists.

As you will find in any book on epidemiology, there are two kinds of problems with reliability. One is random error. Random error will drive associations towards zero. However, with random error, enough numbers can overcome this problem. The other kind of error is systematic error, where one reader reads more positively than another reader, e.g., at two different centers. Unless there is careful assessment of comparability, it is very difficult to be sure — when a difference in rates across centers occurs — whether this is a true difference in the populations or due to differences in readers. To be frank, I'm not sure if this problem has been adequately tackled by the MICOL group. There are reliability data, however I am not sure that as collected they give a good grasp of how a reader in one center compares with a a reader in another, and whether or not there is systematic error. Especially since this is the primary end point of the study, I urge that the problem be rigorously addressed, so as not to compromise what is potentially the most important study on the epidemiology of gallstones at the present time.

As to the independent variables, the exposures, there is a related point which ought to be made. In my judgment, one of the key exposures — in terms of disturbances in human culture that could be contributing to gall-stones — is the nutritional exposure, and by this I mean not just caloric balance.

Caloric balance is easy to assess — people are weighed, height is measured, girth, skinfolds, hip to waist ratios, etc. More difficult is the composition of the diet — total fat, saturated fat, monounsaturated fat, polyunsaturated (omega 6, omega 3) fat, dietary cholesterol, carbohydrate (simple, complex), etc. To get good nutritional data is expensive, particularly on individuals, so that people within a population can be classified without too much error. The short-list food frequency method is probably not adequate for this purpose. A single 24-hr recall is also of limited reliability since in most of our societies people vary much in eating pattern from day to day. With a single 24-hr recall, there is a high ratio of intra- to inter-individual variation and considerable mis-classification on all variables. Thus the results of one recall are compromised — if one puts poor data into the computer, one gets poor data out, no matter how sophisticated the statistical tools used. The epidemiology of hypertension, of gallstones, of cancer need good nutritional data. These do not so far exist and we must not allow ourselves to be intimidated by issues of cost into satisfying ourselves with anything less than good data. Their collection is in the long run truly economical, in terms of cost effectiveness — getting valid research answers to big key questions.

As a colleague of mine recently said, so you have six within-population studies, done with an inadequate nutritional method, all of which show no relationship between dietary lipid and breast cancer — six studies in which everyone consistently concludes there is no relationship. What we have in essence are six false negative studies. And what has been accomplished? Short-list food frequency methods are usually limited and inadequate for characterizing individuals in regard to many nutrients, including dietary lipids.

In this regard, I would like at this point to underscore a concept that took us a long time to learn, as we had to do so in the face of the resistance of another idea. The concept is that dietary constituents, among them dietary fats, including cholesterol, can influence disease over and above their effect on blood constituents, e.g., serum lipids. In the coronary field many of us assumed for years that dietary lipids are important because — and only because — they influence serum cholesterol. But we've also learned slowly and painfully, now that the data are extensive on this question, that dietary cholesterol for example, relates to risk over and above — independent of and additive to — its effect on serum total cholesterol.

In the gallstones field it would seem wise to consider dietary factors possibly influencing gallstone risk in multivariate models to explore whether — in addition to their effects on other constituents, e.g., blood lipids, bile lipids — dietary factors are significant independent exposures. I deem this to be likely. Thus, gallstones are rare in Japan compared to other industrialized countries. Probably this is due to traditional differences in the Japanese diet. This is all part of the same complex — breast cancer, gallstones, colon cancer, coronary disease are all comparatively rare in Japan, but gastric cancer is common. This has little to do with ethnicity or population genetics. After two generations in the United States, everything changes and those of Japanese origin are just about as susceptible as any other American group to these problems. Thus nutritional constituents, in addition to influencing many commonly measured intermediate biomedical variables related to mechanisms, may well have an independent effect over and above other traits which are usually easier to measure. Surely those dietary effects operate through various pathophysiological pathways, but it should not be assumed that these are just the ones usually measured.

Now that I have covered some methodological and conceptual issues, I would like to deal with the question of prevention and put on the table an isssue not on the agenda of this meeting but which, I hope, will be on the agenda of the next. Are we now in a position, based on present knowledge, to do something about the prevention of gallstones? Can we tackle those exposures about which we know enough, so that we can, with some confidence, speak about intervention, confident that the benefits are sizable and the risks small? I believe that there are possibilities now.

First and foremost there is the matter of obesity and gallstones. Nowadays, given modern life styles, imbalances are frequent between energy consumption and energy output, leading to the development of obesity. This is a serious problem in 'western' industrialized societies, even among children and from young adulthood on. This problem must be addressed first of all at the level of primary prevention, not just at the level of treatment for fat people. The main challenge is to prevent the evolution in the population of life style patterns which, year after year, for youth and young adults, lead to a majority becoming more obese.

This I say against a background of self-criticism. In the United States we have accomplished much with regard to improving life styles. We have influenced the composition of the diet — less saturated fat, less cholesterol, and serum lipids have been reduced as a consequence. We have influenced smoking habits. We have influenced the amount of exercise by the population. However, we have had no favorable influence at all on body weight, except among a small stratum of the most educated and affluent who have registered a slight decrease in degree of overweight. In fact, in our country,

mean body mass index of young adults in the three national surveys —
1960—62, the early 70's, and the late 70's — has progressively increased.
This is clearly a challenging problem, not adequately addressed to date by
medical care and public health. This has left the field wide open to all kinds
of commercial, profit making operations that are unsatisfactory. Obesity is a
problem of the modern world. Very soon the Japanese, the Chinese will in all
likelihood also experience it. Before this situation deteriorates any further we
must come to grips with it. In my view what is needed is a proper mix of
better nutrition and exercise from childhood on, for primary prevention
above all; both of these could be important in preventing gallstone disease.

More has to be done, too, on the treatment of already obese people,
particularly with practical diets — not drastic reductions to 500 calories a
day, but modest caloric restrictions with the goal of gradual weight loss
sustained over a long period and then a conscious effort to retain that weight
loss by adoption permanently of better eating and exercise habits. This is the
key challenge, as we all know.

Such an approach could form part of the prevention of gallstones, as well
as the prevention and treatment of hypertension, hyperlipidemia, diabetes,
gout, etc.

This leads me to the question of triglycerides. High triglycerides are highly
responsive, in the overwhelming majority of cases, to weight loss with a
fat-modified diet. Therefore any diet which includes reduction in total fat can
be helpful. I would sound a note of warning against drug approaches to the
triglyceride question as a means of preventing gallstone disease. We only
have to look at the clofibrate experience. Clofibrate is a magnificent drug for
lowering triglycerides, but it produces gallstones!

What about HDL cholesterol, which is inversely related to gallstone risk in
a number of studies? Weight reduction, cessation of smoking, and increased
exercise all tend to raise HDL levels, and merit vigorous pursuit. But I would
not recommend alcohol consumption either as an approach to preventing
coronary disease or gallstone disease. There are enough personal and societal
problems already with regard to excess alcohol consumption.

We can do much through medical care and public health to improve life
styles — diet composition, weight control, exercise, smoking cessation, and
simultaneously do something about triglycerides and HDL cholesterol in a
safe way, all with the potential to prevent gallstone disease.

Nor should we forget the serum cholesterol issue and a possible inverse
relationship with gallstones. An inverse relationship has also been a source of
difficulty with regard to the cancer question, since in some studies those with
very low serum cholesterol have a higher risk of cancer. However, it should
be pointed out that all the epidemiological data are purely observational,
dealing with people — rare and unusual people — observed to have very low
cholesterol. No data exist on the question: by improving diet, taking the best
of Mediterranean and Far East patterns to lower serum cholesterol, does this
have any adverse effect on risk of cancer or gallstone disease? Looking at

Japan and its low gallstone rate, I doubt it. Hence my advice is to implement those diets which are being recommended in Italy, in the U.S.A., and in other countries to prevent coronary disease. Particularly with attention to caloric balance, those also may well have the potential to prevent gallstones. This can be done with only minimal concern for risks with regard to what happens to serum cholesterol although we, as epidemiologists, have to monitor this question.

Finally, let us take a brief look at social class. In many countries with mass problems of coronary and cardiovascular disease, and of high blood pressure, the lower the social class nowadays the bigger the risks. This is probably true for gallstones as well. Obesity in many of our societies is now very common among less affluent, less educated people, both men and women. Moreover, such women also tend to have more children, which is a clear risk factor for gallstone disease. Hence, attention must be given to the social class issue in developing strategies of prevention of gallstone disease. I would urge the MICOL Study to look at this question very carefully, controlling for other factors in the cross-sectional data and ultimately in the prospective data.

Systematic trials are in order on prevention. Nowadays, with sonography available, huge sample size is not necessary nor is excessively long-term follow-up, to assess ability to prevent gallstones. Randomized controlled trials should be put on the agenda, with designs involving working with one group intensely and allowing another group to go its usual way. Public health recommendations can and should be made while developing and conducting trials to accrue special experience and learn in greater detail what actually happens.

Index

Developments in Gastroenterology

1. A. S. Peña, I.T. Weterman, C.C. Booth and W. Strober (eds.): *Recent Advances in Crohn's Disease.* Proceedings of the 2nd International Workshop on Crohn's Disease, held in Noordwijk/Leiden, The Netherlands (1980). 1981   ISBN 90–247–2475–9

2. P.M. Motta and L.J.A. Didio (eds.): *Basic and Clinical Hepatology.* 1982
ISBN 90–247–2404–X

3. D. Rachmilewitz (ed.): *Inflammatory Bowel Diseases.* Proceedings of the 1st International Symposium, held in Jerusalem, Israel (1981). 1982   ISBN 90–247–2612–3

4. D. Fleischer, D. Jensen and P. Bright-Asare (eds.): *Therapeutic Laser Endoscopy in Gastrointestinal Disease.* 1983   ISBN 0–89838–577–6

5. S.P. Borriello (ed.): *Antibiotic Associated Diarrhoea and Colitis.* The Role of *Clostridium difficile* in Gastrointestinal Disorders. 1984   ISBN 0–89838–623–3

6. Ch.H. Gips and R.A.F. Krom (eds.): *Progress in Liver Transplantation.* 1985
ISBN 0–89838–726–4

7. G.F. Nelis, J. Boevé and J.J. Misiewicz (eds.): *Peptic Ulcer Disease: Basic and Clinical Aspects.* Proceedings of a Symposium on Peptic Ulcer Today, held at the Sophia Ziekenhuis, Zwolle, The Netherlands (1984). 1985   ISBN 0–89838–759–0

8. D. Rachmilewitz (ed.): *Inflammatory Bowel Diseases 1986.* Proceedings of the 2nd International Symposium, held in Jerusalem, Israel (1985). 1986   ISBN 0–89838–796–5

9. E.M.H. Mathus-Vliegen: *The Role of Laser in Gastroenterology.* Analysis of Eight Years' Experience. 1989   ISBN 0–7923–0425–X

10. D.M. Jensen and J.-M. Brunetaud (eds.): *Medical Laser Endoscopy.* 1990
ISBN 0–7923–0579–5

11. D. Rachmilewitz and J. Zimmerman (eds.): *Inflammatory Bowel Diseases 1990.* Proceedings of the 3rd International Symposium, held in Jerusalem, Israel (1989). 1990
ISBN 0–7923–0657–0

12. L. Capocaccia, G. Ricci, F. Angelico, M. Angelico, A.F. Attili and L. Lalloni (eds.): *Recent Advances in the Epidemiology and Prevention of Gallstone Disease.* Proceedings of the 2nd International Workshop, held in Rome, Italy (1989). 1991   ISBN 0-7923-0994-4

Kluwer Academic Publishers – Dordrecht / Boston / London